THE STRONG ONES

How a Band of Civilian Women Made Their Mark on the Army

SARA HAMMEL

Published by SARA HAMMEL

For information, address sarahammelbooks@gmail.com

www.sarahammelbooks.com

Cover design by Rocking Book Covers
Cover photo copyright © Sara Hammel. Left to right: Nadine, Sara, Laurie, Marion, unnamed volunteer 1, unnamed volunteer 2
Formatting by Polgarus Studio

For the women of the Natick strength study—
and for everyone facing their own Cement Hill. Never give up.

Contents

Author's note

Dozens of us went through one special Army study, but each individual—test subjects, scientists, trainers and interns—experienced it differently. This story has been told with the help of many others who were there, but the tale is filtered through my eyes, and I never mean to speak for everyone. There were test subjects I couldn't find, some who never responded, and some who declined to participate in the book. My experience in 1995 might differ greatly from theirs; their stories are their own, as are their personal beliefs. Any political opinions or statements within this work are solely mine unless otherwise noted.

I used diaries, newspaper articles and dozens of interviews to accurately report past events. Our memories didn't always match, and I have taken some literary license in recounting some moments. For privacy reasons, some names and details have been changed, and there are a (very) few composite characters. And finally, the women of the Natick strength study were never soldiers. Few of us had experience with the military ourselves or through our families. We were civilians treading on unfamiliar ground, and we were honored to carry water for the women doing the work of defending our country. I want to thank our servicewomen and men, veterans, and their families for their service. I write here about painful blisters and tough backpack treks, but members of our armed forces face trials far greater and that's not something I take lightly.

I wrote this book for those who went through the study to say, *We were here*. It is a book for and about ordinary people doing extraordinary things. For many of us, the study remains one of the most important and amazing things we ever did. The test subjects did our small part in one moment in time, and I have tried to honor that.

"When men restrict who can fight and die for America, they restrict who can run America." — *Arie Taylor, the first Black noncommissioned officer in charge of women's Air Force training.*

And though she be but little, she is fierce.
—from A Midsummer Night's Dream by William Shakespeare

Prologue

In the summer of 2018, as the United States Marine Corps (USMC) was celebrating 100 years of women in its ranks, twenty-two-year-old Second Lieutenant Catherine Afton was at Quantico learning how to be a leader. She'd already studied the history of women in the Corps, and that summer she absorbed more of it, wrapped as it was in a package of energy and excitement about the centennial. On rare breaks in her training, she volunteered to help create inspirational social media content to shine a light on the life of Opha May Johnson, the first woman ever to enlist. Every Marine knows who Johnson is; enough of them have answered the call of "First female Marine!" from drill instructors and shouted back, "Ma'm, the first female Marine was Opha May Johnson, ma'am!"

Catherine was no exception—she knew all about the legend. Johnson enlisted as World War I was nearing its end, a time when men were needed to fight overseas and there were clerical roles to fill back home. When the Corps asked women to step in and help out, Johnson accepted the challenge and made it to the front of the line ahead of some

300 other women who wanted to serve. When she was sworn in at age forty on August 13, 1918, officials had to cross out the male pronouns on her official enlistment paper.

Catherine Afton had never dreamed of joining up—hers is not a military family. But the Marine ethos was naturally strong in her. Almost from birth, she wanted to be the best at anything and everything. How Catherine came to be at Quantico that summer is part of this story. Her world is entwined with that of the women of the Natick strength study as inextricably as our story is entrenched in Army history. It was a matter of fierce ambition and a stroke of fate that drew Catherine in and put her where she was meant to be, setting her down in the perfect place at the exact right time. Her career prospects were wide open in a way they never were for so many women in the past—she could join the infantry, potentially lead a platoon into combat, even switch branches and attempt to become a Navy SEAL if she wanted to.

That summer, while she was paying homage to strong women who came before her, she was standing on the shoulders of those very people. Those who risked their lives. Gave their lives. Fought for our country. Gathered intelligence. Never gave up. Those who performed in all the smaller ways and with a general badassery that, when added up over time, can change the world.

Catherine knew that Opha May Johnson broke down that first barrier in the Marines, but women in every branch of the military—and out of it—have also done their part.

For centuries women were banned from combat roles, paid less than men and denied promotions, yet there are endless stories of women rising up and taking their place after they were told *no*. Some bravely ran toward peril and paid with their lives. Did Catherine know that Army wife Molly Pitcher took up arms to fend off charging Redcoats in the Revolutionary War, or that Sarah Edmonds made the ultimate sacrifice in the Civil War, fighting and dying disguised as Union solider Frank Thompson? Had she heard about Cathay Williams, who, when she joined up as "William Cathay" in 1866, became the first documented Black woman to enlist in the Army?

In 1989, Army Captain Linda Bray would be the first woman to lead a combat mission in this country's history, even as the law said she wasn't allowed to fight.

There was Four-star Admiral Michelle Howard, who became the highest-ranking Black woman in Navy history when she was sworn in as Vice Chief of Naval Operations in 2014.

There was Major General Jeannie Marie Leavitt, who flew higher, further, faster as the first female fighter pilot for the U.S. Air Force.

And there was us, with a contribution perhaps smaller but made with iron will and mighty hearts nonetheless, for the Army.

PART ONE

YOU GOTTA BE

1

You gotta be

May 1995

There is a certain kind of woman who lives to work out. She crams exercise into her day at the expense of sleep, chases endorphins like a surfer chases waves, climbs mountains, competes in mud runs, flips tractor tires. Maybe she joins the military to make a career of it.

We were not those women. The forty-five civilian volunteers of the Army strength study taking place on a base in Massachusetts that year were, by and large, recently off the couch, lapsed college athletes, occasional joggers or sometime observers of sport who set forth to do something extraordinary, and as they signed their names to the human test subject agreement thought, *Maybe it's my turn. Maybe this is my one shot to find out what I'm made of. I'm going to help change the world—watch me.*

When the experiment first began, I stood on the edge of the wood with six other women I barely knew, wobbling under the weight of my 75-pound pack as we waited for the *go* signal. The volunteers—all civilians save for one—had been divided into four training groups for the seven-month trial. I was assigned to C-Group, a ragtag assortment of test subjects who trained every day at one-thirty.

I stared down a wooded path with steep hills and sharp bends, impossibly narrow in parts and strewn with hazards of rocks and roots, kicked the dust into dirty clouds, felt the vibration in the soles of my feet. I was nervously blurting unhelpful things: *My feet already hurt. This doesn't look that hard. This pack is pulling me down. I like your boots.* I kept an eye on our trainer Eric Lammi, blond and six-three and wryly, uproariously funny, except when he wielded his dreaded stopwatch and needed us to perform. There was nothing amusing to him about our scores, our times, our training. An Olympic trials-caliber decathlete did not become that by getting distracted by life's frivolities, worrying whether he was liked, or by coddling anyone.

Nadine was there, standing near me if not next to me, her shoulder-length chestnut curls held back by a lilac headband tied with a bow. She strode to the start line with careful examination, a quiet way about her, and curious brown eyes. Elle, still the most authentically positive woman I ever met, flanked my other side. The study's one soldier, Private First Class Marion Cavanaugh, always quietly did her job and waited on the fringes.

I looped my thumbs under my shoulder straps as Eric

offered one final tip before sending us on our way. "You'll walk, shuffle, jog, run—whatever gets you to the finish line fastest," he told us. *Run*? With this thing on? *Don't fall on your ass,* I thought. *Don't break your teeth on a rock and have to claw your way home through the dirt.* "Your times today will set the stage for the next seven months."

The pack's belt dug into my waist. My boots weren't broken in yet. I was uncomfortable in my skin as a civilian invading a severe, imposing military world, and I'd felt like an interloper the moment I'd driven my car past the Army base's drab, gray buildings and walked their halls for the first time. I was twenty-four and trying to dodge mediocrity like it was a missile aimed dead at me. As adulthood stretched ahead of me as wide as a continent, I knew I was supposed to gaze across and see marriage, kids and the ultimate prize in the distance—settling down. A successful career was a nice bonus, but the one thing a woman must have, the societal requirement for a well-lived life, is your own family. But the thought of such ordinariness gave me hives. I craved freedom and adventure.

Elle, a stay-at-home mom, smiled through obvious jitters. They said we couldn't do it, so we knew we must. Eric hit his timer and yelled for us to *Go, go, go!* We took our first steps in the journey to change our bodies—and maybe the world. My legs were leaden and my boot scraped the ground as I walked; I was as nimble as a glacier. The pack pressed on my back, my lungs, my shoulders. A smaller woman next to me was panting and falling behind. The backpack was two-thirds of her body weight.

Everything about the scene screamed underdogs, outliers, insanity. They called us ordinary, and on paper perhaps we were: Teachers, stay-at-home moms, working moms, bartenders, beauticians, lawyers, a landscaper, a prison guard and one reporter had joined up. Some women hadn't been to a gym…ever. Some struggled to jog a mile *without* a backpack. Some were not much heavier than the packs they were carrying.

That day in the woods I stumbled and just barely stopped myself from going flying. And then a voice blasted through the spring air and echoed in the wood. "You can do it. Come on! Don't give up. We're in this together." It was Elle again. *We're in this together.* Oh, so I wasn't alone, even though I felt like it for brief moments when my insecurities swarmed me like killer bees. That day, I kept going. I was in those woods trying to change the world in my own small way, as were many of the test subjects who'd taken over a patch of this Army base for an experiment whose goal was simple on its face: To determine if women could get strong enough to succeed at the toughest military jobs usually assigned to men. We were stand-ins for female soldiers who were busy doing the work of defending our country.

Simple as the study's stated goal was, it carried with it a long history of sexism, politics and controversy, and it had already attracted the attention of powerful people in Washington—mostly politicians and conservative pundits, mostly male—who'd tried to halt it before it could start. And so that day, gutting it out in those woods, we bore a weight greater than the hunks of metal in our packs.

No one was sure where it would lead. No one knew whether this attempt would explode or fizzle out like faulty fireworks, if we would stay the course as we pushed our bodies past their limits or if we would fail military women—or *all* women. What had we gotten ourselves into? And who in their right minds would sign *us* up for something like this? Who would risk looking like fools by taking a political hot potato and passing it off to a bunch of untrained, untested civilians?

January 1995

The new year blew in clear and cold in Massachusetts, stinging exposed faces and hands with a series of zero-degree days. From their offices at the U.S. Army Research Institute of Environmental Medicine (USARIEM) on the U.S. Army Soldier Systems Command (USASSC) base in Natick, Mass., research scientists Everett Harman and Pete Frykman were readying their latest study. Their proposal to investigate the physical potential of female soldiers had attracted ample funding, and space for a custom gym on the base was reserved for a March start. Now it was time to recruit the all-important test subjects—and two top-notch trainers to help guide them.

The two research physiologists, who first struck up a friendship in graduate school at the University of Massachusetts at Amherst in the early eighties, had spent the last decade innovating and problem-solving to build a stronger, more lethal soldier. They'd each done important work for the U.S. military, though the average person might not realize it based on such unglamorous report titles as "Quantitation of progressive muscle fatigue during dynamic leg exercise in humans" and "Anthropometric Correlates of Maximal Locomotion Speed Under Heavy Backpack Loads."

The experiment they were planning for that spring had an equally long, dry moniker: "Effects of a specifically designed conditioning program on the load carriage and lifting performance of female soldiers." Abstruse title or not, this one was special. One word in particular would set it apart from many of the studies the Army had sponsored over the years: "female." Though women have been serving in the U.S. military—officially and unofficially—for centuries, their unique physical capabilities hadn't been thoroughly and exhaustively examined.

That needed to change. Women made up about 14 percent of the U.S. military and their numbers were growing. They were soldiers, officers, Marines, sailors, medics and much, much more. Many of them served in MOSs (military occupational specialties, or "jobs" in civilian-speak) that required significant upper-body strength. But without proper physical training, a high proportion of women found it difficult to manage the toughest aspects of those roles. Basic Training, the entrance course that teaches skills like handling a weapon, teamwork and general physical fitness, was never enough to strengthen the right muscles and only improved female recruits' lifting capacity by 8 to 12 percent. There had to be another way.

Enter Everett and Pete. They hypothesized that "the ability of women to perform heavy physical tasks in the U.S. Army could be greatly improved by having them engage in a specially designed and professionally administered physical training program, under normal Army time constraints." In other words, they wanted to devise an efficient, targeted workout regimen that would help female soldiers excel in the toughest jobs. Some of those roles were in combat, but many were everyday positions women have held through the ages.

As Pete explained, "For a light-wheel vehicle mechanic on a non-armored vehicle, changing a 140-pound Humvee tire is a one-person job. And oddly enough, cooks have to be strong. People who are cooks handle huge amounts of food in an industrial kitchen. Hundred-gallon batches are physically demanding. It's not like a cup of this and a pinch of that. It's fifty pounds of potatoes."

The two scientists had always known how tough women are. They'd seen the strongest among them outperform men in the physical arena inside and out of the military. But the fact remained that on average, females possess around 50 to 60 percent of males' upper body strength. And so Everett, fifty-one, an earnest, thoughtful man with a Ph.D. in exercise science, was ready to chart a course around nature. After years of observing the unique skills of both male and female soldiers, it was increasingly obvious to him that women were being underestimated and could do more than people tended to expect of them. He comes from a family of fascinating females—he is the son of a school administrator, brother of a pulmonary and intensive care hospital physician, and nephew of an avocado rancher and expert in rare citrus fruits—and was baffled by a world that didn't comprehend the power of women. "I never knew any different," Everett would say when the question was posed to him. "The least accomplished person in my family is a man. I wasn't as aware of discrimination; I never looked at it in quantitative terms."

The time had come. As the principal investigator on this new study, Everett had proposed and designed the intricately punishing regimen his volunteers would endure for months. He prescribed twenty-four weeks of rigorous physical workouts to include lifting heavy boxes and weights, running, 75-pound backpack marches, and 110-pound trailer pulls over mixed terrain. In between all that would be three testing phases to take place at the beginning, middle and end of the experiment. Everett and Pete calculated they'd need at least twenty female soldiers to ensure valid results, a number that accounted for expected attrition and pregnancy (which would require mandatory withdrawal). In the end they decided to try for forty subjects to make the findings still more valid.

The experiment would be groundbreaking in important ways. First, as Everett wrote in a report about the study, "there has been little research on the effects of physical conditioning programs on the physical work capacity of women." Furthermore, he explained, "Women have been minimally tested as to their ability to carry heavy backpack loads." Lugging supplies and equipment on foot is a vital function of military ground forces, and soldiers regardless of gender should to be able to do it at sustained speed and distances. Everett and Pete's research on backpack loads, therefore, was poised to become some of the most advanced of its time.

Women have long played a vital role in our nation's defenses, but were never equal members of our military. They couldn't reap the same benefits as men thanks to the 1948 Women's Armed Services Integration Act, which effectively banned them from direct combat roles—which is where the prized medals, promotions and pay are earned. This ban remained until 1994, when a new twist on the rule came into force. That fresh, updated policy was touted as a way to open more doors for women, and technically it did: The Department of Defense (DOD) would now allow certain exceptions for *some* females to be in combat under *some* circumstances. But they were still effectively excluded from direct combat and infantry and would continue to be kept out of MOSs in which "job-related physical requirements would exclude the vast majority of women."

The reasons given for these ongoing policies were less than compelling. At a 1994 press briefing, officials explained that the DOD believed the assignment of women to direct ground combat units "would not contribute to the readiness and effectiveness of those units" because of physical strength, stamina, and privacy issues, that neither the public nor

Congress wanted it, and that there were enough men available to do the fighting so women weren't needed. Women still could not even attempt to qualify for some 221,000 of the military's 1.4 million available positions.

But there were always people lobbying for those discriminatory policies to be peeled away entirely. Rep. Patricia Schroeder, a Democrat from Colorado with a seat on the influential House Armed Services Committee, had been fighting for equality for decades. She'd worked tirelessly to force military academies including West Point to admit women in the seventies, and in the nineties she championed a $40 million appropriation for the Defense Women's Health Research Program (DWHRP), a grant package created to fund studies into a spectrum of issues affecting military women's bodies and minds. When Everett learned about this brand-new program, he pounced.

"I always knew women could do it. But the opportunity hadn't arisen for me to do something like this study until that grant money," Everett explained. "We applied—a lot of people applied—and we got a lot of money for equipment and things." He received $140,000 from the DWHRP to prove his hypothesis, and once he set his mind to something like this, watch out. One colleague described him as "one of the smartest people I've ever met. He takes in data at an unbelievable rate. He is incredibly clear-eyed."

By the winter of 1995, everything was falling into place for a March start for the scientists' audacious attempt—everything, that is, except for the most crucial element of all: the human test subjects.

Everett finished a phone call, pulled on his jacket and grabbed his gym bag. He strode out of the office and set off apace, taking the long way past frigid Lake Cochituate covered in sheets of grey ice. He came across soldiers running in formation, heard them belt out the cadence call that made their labor more bearable, then wound around a bend in the road toward the base's gym. Everett didn't simply study the biomechanics of the human form—physical fitness and performance were his life, too, and his claim to fame was his ability to bench-press over 300 pounds, a substantial heft by any measure.

Before he hit the weight room, he stopped at one of the Labs' public areas to check the bulletin board. The base had one central location where the soldiers who were available to act as test subjects were listed, and any current study looking for volunteers drew from the same batch. Everett found the list of people on the base who were free to do a seven-month experiment and ran his finger down the ladder of names, which was lengthy enough, bursting with volunteers who were ready to help further military research. He scanned every line. Then he read it all again. One female name jumped out at him from a litany of *Johns, Mikes* and *Bobs*: *Private First Class Marion Cavanaugh*. One woman was available. *One*.

It was never easy to find large numbers of female soldiers who could leave their posts for any extended period of time, and Everett's study would be no different. Exacerbating things was the very appropriation that had blessed him with his funding: Thanks to the DWHRP money, studies on women were sprouting up throughout the military, including at the Natick base, draining the volunteer pool until it was shallower than ever.

The military cannot innovate without human test subjects. Without us, scientists can't develop the most efficient nutrition for long marches, study altitude sickness to prepare for mountainous missions, or tackle heat stroke so soldiers can function optimally in the desert. The historically sinister aspects of government-sponsored studies like the infamous Tuskegee Syphilis Experiment—in which hundreds of Black men with syphilis were lured by the Public Health Service with free meals and health care, weren't told they were ill, and weren't treated—were supposed to be over, and in fact the abomination that caused the death of dozens of men also led to the creation of the Office for Human Research Protections (OHRP) along with new federal laws protecting human subjects. The strength study test subjects, then, could expect to be in safe, capable hands.

The Natick base was ground zero for cutting-edge military research. Known colloquially as the Labs, the sprawling property hums with possibility. Strolling through its labyrinthine roads and walkways gives the sense of potential breakthroughs simmering just beneath the surface. Anything an American warfighter wears, carries or eats comes from the Labs, which opened in 1954 with a remit to build a better, stronger, more lethal soldier. Scientists on the product and gadget side have developed a vest pocket that pipes liquid nutrition straight to the mouth of a soldier on the move, a space-age metallic covering for desert camouflage, freeze-dried salads, and radioactive cockroaches that ended up running amok in Natick in the 1970s. There have been rumors of "courage pills" being studied, and the base boasts climatic chambers that can dip to seventy below zero with 40 m.p.h. winds, rain or even snow. Their scientists are credited with the invention of chicken nuggets and, in one later development they called "the Holy Grail," a pizza—one of the most-requested meals by soldiers in the field—with a *three-year* shelf life.

Everett and Pete worked for the medical and environmental side. USARIEM studies health and performance and the impact of environmental stressors on soldiers, including anything related to nutrition, exercise, heat and cold. Pete, forty-three, bespectacled and a keen rollerblader, explained that while the details of each research journey vary, the basic goal is the same: "Even your study wasn't so much about, can we make these *women* strong?" He told me of the new study that year. "The question is always: how can we make *soldiers* more lethal and more survivable so they can do their soldiering job better?"

The Army kept a rotating pool of soldiers whose main job was to act as test subjects, and Marion Cavanaugh was one of them. She and a handful of other medics had been plucked from training at an Army base in San Antonio in 1994 and offered a unique opportunity up in Massachusetts. "Every time there was a study with human subjects, they would do a briefing with us—and it was totally up to us whether to volunteer," Marion, then a few months shy of her twentieth birthday, told me of her new job on the Natick base. "There had to be full disclosure and we'd have to sign documents. We were always free to quit at any time with no repercussions."

She agreed to be run off her feet, poked, prodded and dressed up in the name of science. Some experiments needed her for a week, some for a day, others for an hour or two. One gig had her trying on body armor designed for female fighter pilots. "I had to wear the body armor and show them how I could reach to the left and to the right. They were testing my range of motion," she explained.

By the winter of 1995, Marion hadn't yet faced anything particularly onerous on the job though she was pushing herself hard on the fitness front. She'd wake up when it was still dark, wrap her long auburn hair into a low bun, and head out for PT. The esprit de corps was robust on the small base, and on the days drill instructors threw in a 10-mile run, passersby could hear the soldiers' footfall between the call and answer of their work song. At night Marion would often accompany her boyfriend, Private First Class Billy Wade—another medic she met at San Antonio—to the gym. While he practiced taekwondo, she'd tackle cardio and weight training. When she was approached by her superiors about the upcoming strength study that would need her for a full seven months, she listened to the briefing and thought, *More working out? Sign me up.*

Marion was young, strong, and eager, but she couldn't take on the new study alone. The news that the Army would provide Everett and Pete with *one* female soldier was not entirely shocking but it was a blow nonetheless. In some smaller, less involved experiments, turning to civilians wouldn't have been a problem, or even particularly unusual. But for this kind of commitment and intensity, recruiting and retaining the average woman would be an unusual challenge. Especially, says Everett, because they had a little extra grant money available to attract quality subjects, but due to certain stipulations, "we weren't allowed to spend it on recruiting."

Everett and Pete pivoted to a free and effective way of attracting subjects: a media blitz. They contacted Boston TV stations and sent out a press release to local newspapers. They offered $500 upon completion of the study and highlighted the personal training aspect of the experiment. They sugarcoated nothing in their zeal to attract viable subjects, laying out exactly how rigorous it would be. And then they waited to see who would be courageous—or foolish—enough to respond.

One town away, I was working as a reporter for the *Middlesex News*, a mid-sized daily paper that covered around a dozen towns in the MetroWest area of Massachusetts. No day was the same in the suburbs. There were sewer committee meetings, raccoons in the rubbish, sometimes a stabbing, an occasional mysterious crime and a smattering of stories about ordinary citizens doing extraordinary things. At night I'd hit the town with the paper's pack of ambitious young journalists, a cadre of dreamers who spent evenings talking over beers about our beats and where we wanted to end up, which was rarely where we were.

I packed in my exercise before work, setting out in the frigid winter dawn four mornings a week, scraping the frost off my car and driving to Walden Pond. Around the time Everett and Pete put out their press release I was out at seven a.m. hiking past the barren oaks and mighty pines thickening those legendary woods. I ran, stretched my legs, felt the cold air stabbing my lungs like a thousand little daggers, and raised the volume on my yellow Walkman. I went there to blend in with the trees and to escape the glare of fitter, thinner gym-goers. In Walden Woods only nature and the occasional early-morning hiker bore witness to my plodding imperfections.

I hit an incline and waited for the whisper runners swear they hear: *Keep going. You're free. Run!* A different tune was blowing in my ear: *Stop immediately. This is too hard.* I did, then checked my watch. Less than four minutes this time, a.k.a. most of Des'ree's hit song *You Gotta Be*, which meant today's attempt changed nothing; I still loathed running. I didn't like the pounding on my joints and the vibrations through my bones.

I hiked another fifty feet until I came upon Thoreau's ruins. What had been the transcendentalist's home of a century and a half ago was gone and marked now by granite posts and crumbling stones with a dusting of snow in the crevices. I'd read *Walden; or, life in the woods*, and I *got* the satire in it and Henry David Thoreau's idea of nature as divine. I related to the idea of escaping, of hiding and writing and taking myself out of the cruel, prickly world for a while; this place was a gift for introverts to retreat to when our minds descended into chaos. I waited for inspiration from the spirit of the late philosopher, but none came, so I took off on a fast walk.

It was a confounding thing, this inability to run. I'd grown up hanging out at a health club owned by my father and started playing tennis seriously at age fourteen, did the sprints they asked of me (coming in last most times unless I cheated), and ended up ranked in the top 20 in New England for girls eighteen and under. But there was something about the particular pain of distance that my mind and body found intolerable. Instead of a runner's high, I was overcome with jogger's irritability. These repeated failures fuelled my determination to find the joy in it, and to somehow join that special club of fit and happy and thin people. After one more lap around the pond, I headed back to my car. If it wasn't snowing, I'd be back to try again tomorrow.

After a hurried shower I made my first visit of the day to an addictive New England institution we'll call Donut Depot. When they asked me after I ordered one of their wicked good coffees, *Anything else?* I took a moment, as I always did, to listen to the voice that's tried to save me my whole life but rarely gets her fair due: *You don't need sugar. You do not want junk food.*

"No, thank you," I said to the nice lady trying to push frosted cinnamon buns on me. *Not today, Satan.* I drove to work with my French vanilla coffee knowing the fight would go on; there would be infinite encounters with temptation at that place, and always another chance to give in. I remember one visit to Donut Depot after I was sent to cover a bomb scare at a supermarket. I'd raced to the scene, examined everything as best I could from outside the yellow tape, then found the lieutenant in charge. Notebook out, pen poised over the page, long summer dress reaching my ankles and covering my chest, I asked for details about the potential crime scene.

Unbutton your dress first. Then I'll give you the information, the cop leered. I'd always rather laugh off dirtbags than go back to my editor without a story, so I rolled my eyes through humiliation and disgust. Donut Depot was across the street. On the way back to the office to file my story about a "bomb" that turned out to be a paper bag, I ate two-and-a-half donuts (always leave something behind as tangible proof of restraint). I did it because the sugar sedated me, but also because it distracted me. Suddenly I felt bad about the calories, not the harassment. Donuts and their ilk were my shield, my weapon, my fortress and my retreat.

I got to work and settled at my desk in the bustling newsroom, downing coffee and cruising the wires with no inkling my life was about to change. I saw the *Middlesex News's* well-respected metro editor out of the corner of my eye. Jan Gardner was one of the toughest editors I ever had, and right then she was making a beeline for my desk. She approached, laid the Local section of that day's newspaper in front of me, and pointed to an unassuming story. I read it, and I was baffled. It was a call for civilian volunteers to join a study of women's strength at a nearby Army base in a town I didn't cover, and included such alarming words as "rigorous," "intense," and "extremely heavy weights." The scientists promised a 110-pound trailer pull through hilly, rocky woods. There would be brutal backpack hikes. This delightful torture would go on for one-and-a-half hours a day, five days a week for six months and change.

Right there, amid blaring police scanners and reporters shouting into their phones, in her even, cool way, Jan dared me to do it.

"I'm thirty-seven—over the cutoff age," she said. "But *you* could do it."

"Could do...what?" I asked her.

"You could apply to be a *volunteer*—and write about it."

I continued to miss the point. Jan wasn't my direct supervisor, so I wasn't sure if she was asking or telling me to sign up for this thing. How could I leave work three hours a day—including travel and showering—and still hunt down and write two stories a day on my own beat?

"I'm not sure—"

"—not *sure*? This could be a big story for us. For you."

Jan pointed out the study was a groundbreaking program designed specifically for females, and that it could be a big national story. I still didn't quite get what this had to do with me, and I offered an insipid response along the lines of *Wow, interesting*, followed by, *Sure, I'll look into it.*

After Jan went back to putting out the next day's paper, the primary thoughts running through my mind were reasons why not:

I don't cover the military.

The Army is a violent institution.

I don't like being ordered around.

Why me? (Neither Jan nor I recall the answer to this).

Then I read the piece more carefully. The scientists welcomed women in "average" shape. Candidates should live locally and be between the ages of eighteen and thirty-two. For the next few days, in between sniffing around for scoops in suburbia, I thought about Jan's proposition. It was a potential national story right in my lap, something an ambitious local reporter would be silly to turn down.

There was no one moment or factor that led me to *yes*, though the decision had something to do with how sick I was of predators and how nice it would be to be able to fight them off (this is not how it works, but being strong is *something*, anyway). A diary entry from that winter reads, *Yesterday I first experienced what sexual harassment is. It struck me like a ton of bricks. I cried a little & felt sick. I've heard worse. But nothing ever made me feel this disgusting. [Older male who was senior to me] leaned over my desk, close, and said, 'in a time of long skirts and short hair, thanks for bucking the trend.' Then walked away. I am so mad I want to hurt him. If he does it again I'll kill him. Anyway, gotta clean my room. Love, Sara.*

I couldn't force myself to run one full loop around Walden Pond, but I could lift things, and I'd played tennis for hours on end in high school and college, and I imagined stern-faced military types would be there to prod me when I wanted to give up. *Seven months.* What if I couldn't hack it? But it could change things for women. It could be a huge story.

It could be the body shakeup I needed. I was flailing after an extreme diet months before had shuttered my metabolism like winter was coming; my body now hoarded every calorie as if preparing for extended hibernation. From January through June of 1994, in a do-or-die attack on the beer-and-pizza weight I'd piled on during my last two years of college, I didn't eat a single bite of food. I didn't chew once (that is, after the nutritionist told me my sugarless gum was possibly hindering my weight loss). There was no breaking that diet. With one hit, one sniff, one bite of potato, my system would go haywire. The doctor-supervised plan allowed five shakes a day totaling 800 calories. If you ate solid food, they'd sniff it on you. If you ate, you wouldn't stop.

I lost more than 60 pounds, just like Oprah did on her liquid diet in 1988, after which she wheeled 67 pounds of animal blubber onto the stage while modeling size ten Calvin Klein jeans. And just like Oprah, I began regaining the weight immediately. As she said years later, "What I didn't know [then] was that my metabolism was shot. Two weeks after I returned to real food, I was up ten pounds." She never fit into those jeans again. I felt her pain. I had Guess jeans in my drawer that no longer buttoned up. Was this Army thing the answer? Was getting strong—not skinny but fit—the way to banish my unhealthy thinking for good?

I went to Jan and told her I was in. "Great," she said. "Now you have to get Andrea on board."

That could be where my brief Army dream died. No

editor of a paper our size—circulation around 35,000 during the week and 45,000 on Sundays—could easily afford to pay a reporter to exercise half the day. Furthermore, the Army isn't known for its eagerness to greenlight media coverage it can't control. But the universe was on my side that week, and I found out quickly our new executive editor was a visionary with no shortage of courage. Andrea Haynes, the first female Editor in Chief of the *Middlesex News*, needed only a short briefing to jump on board. I pointed out women were banned from even *attempting* to qualify for tons of military jobs simply because of our gender, but she already knew; her son was a Marine. "This," Andrea said to me without so much as a blink or an argument, "is interesting. I like when reporters show initiative. Let's see if we can make this work."

I got a firm, slow nod of acceptance that day, like a character in a movie who sets everything in motion and sets the plot spiraling into the unknown: Glory or defeat, victory or catastrophe. Andrea got to work figuring out how the paper could finagle this project while I crafted a letter to the scientists explaining why they should let me in—and why they could trust me to portray them, their study, the United States Army, and my fellow volunteers with intelligence and fairness.

I thought I knew then how important this study was. But as a young, privileged suburban white woman who was as likely to walk on the moon as enlist in the Army, I did not recognize yet how much we were still underestimated, underappreciated and discriminated against. I had Betty

Friedan's *The Feminine Mystique* on my bookshelf and Nan Robertson's *The Girls in the Balcony*, about the fight for equal rights for women at the New York *Times*, on my desk at work. I was still trying to figure out Andrea Dworkin. I was in awe of the strides these activists and their feminist sisters had made, but I thought the battle was largely over. I thought we'd won and that there was only a bit of sweeping up left to do and a few little fires to put out.

The nineties had *felt* fair to me: I came of age in a time of Title IX, girl power, a burgeoning career with plenty of strong female bosses, and no need for a man to pay my way. I thought sexual harassment was a part of life we had to accept and learn to deal with. I thought our power lay in handling it well, not in eradicating it; you might as well try to drain the oceans. I didn't have an appreciation for how the feminism I'd studied left so many behind or that intersectional feminism existed. (The concept developed by activist and lawyer Kimberlé Crenshaw addresses the too-often-overlooked fact that "all inequality is not created equal," which means, to offer just one example, that Black women face the double whammy of racism *and* sexism).

I'd made a name for myself at the college newspaper with a series of scathing articles about the massive gap in funding for women's sports, and been assured I'd done it right when the men's basketball coach—the famous Lefty Driesell—called me personally to yell at me for taking on him and his boys. But my stories trumpeted on the front page of a newspaper was progress in itself, right? Things were moving forward. Weren't they? And finally, I didn't focus on the military women who might one day charge into combat in droves, or the ones who already had, and what would happen to them. I would be going into this study with a blunted, broad, cavewoman's understanding that it *simply wasn't fair.*

After I sent in my application, days, then weeks, went by. I didn't hear a word despite some eager follow-up voicemails. I bit my nails and hung out with the gang at Doo Wops, our local suburban "night club." I put Sheryl Crow's *All I Wanna Do* on repeat and longed to be on Santa Monica Boulevard across from the giant carwash in L.A. that she sang about. I dreamed of sunnier places, of getting away from the tight confines of New England where I felt unseen, trapped and too big for the space. I wanted to stretch my arms in a desert, get lost on a mountain, surround myself with people who didn't know me.

The study could be my ticket to a job with the national media, maybe a glossy magazine or a big-city newspaper. I wanted to interview celebrities for *People* magazine—which had never responded to any resume I'd ever sent them—*and* I wanted to win a Pulitzer for social justice reporting. To me, glamour and grit went hand-in-hand in my chosen career. But the weeks were flying by, and I began to give up hope the Army would consider me—or even notice me. I began to stew on the idea they were busy choosing fitter, stronger test subjects while my application lay wadded up in the garbage, unseen.

2

Strong enough

Mary Desmond stepped out of her car and was instantly hit with an arctic blast of bitter wind. The twenty-five-year-old teacher was already exhausted from a long day of work followed by a trek to Boston for graduate school, and now she had studying to look forward to.

As Mary trudged up the walkway of the two-family Natick home she lived in, she spotted her roommate chatting with their landlord by the front door. Mary greeted them both and then listened as the man, who had also become a friend, talked of his exciting new experiment and how it was about strong women in every sense of the word *strong*.

The man was Everett Harman, the scientist I would come to know as "Ev" because that's what his friends called him. Mary's roommate Lisa was immediately intrigued and asked Ev how she could join. Mary was, as I had been, slightly confused upon first hearing of the study. It took her a moment to absorb what he was saying, and then to acknowledge the odd sense that maybe this was something she could be a part of. And just as it had with me, skepticism followed, nipping at her heels, offering up reasons why not. Mary had scarcely enough energy left to go out at night and maintain a viable social life. There was little motivation, and even less time, available for regular exercise.

"I'm too busy…and I'm in the worst shape of my life," she told them. Mary, who stood around five-seven with freckles dotting her nose and short brown curls atop her head, said she was the heaviest she'd ever been and didn't feel great about her fitness level.

Her roommate, on the other hand, had gone to college on an athletics scholarship and kept up her fitness since graduating; she had no doubts. In the next few days the young women marinated on the idea and calculated how much time they could realistically spare over the next seven months. In the end, Lisa wasn't able to shoehorn the study into her busy schedule. But Mary, after giving it some thought and finding Lisa's enthusiasm contagious, paid Ev a visit and told him she was all in.

That same week, a few miles down Rte. 9 in Waltham, graduate student Jane Crowley was lying on the couch watching the eleven o'clock news and "feeling like a slug," as she put it. The five-foot-nine blonde, in her words, was 118 pounds and "extremely out of shape." She bolted upright when she saw a brief report on Channel 5 calling for civilian test subjects for an Army experiment. Jane, also twenty-five, listened intently and thought, *Did they say* civilians*? I'll get paid to work out? BINGO.* She hadn't been doing much physical activity since college and was ready to get fit again.

She called Everett and Pete the next day. By the time she learned the study would be even harder than the news portrayed, she was already hooked. After answering a few questions and assuring the scientists she was fully committed, she went on to pass an Army doctor's physical, and she was *in*. She found it an awkward thing to explain to her fiancé—then in medical school—and her parents. Her father shrugged and her mother supported her while also letting her know her daughter was "a bit nuts," as Jane told me. Many of us had the same issue with the people in our lives. You say you're in a *study*? Like a physical *room* where you prepare for exams? Are you a guinea pig? Did you give blood? How can a *study*—a dry, dull, possibly frightening surrender of your own will—be anything to undertake in a life, to grasp onto and be able to say of it, *This is one of the best things I will ever do?*

At the exact moment Jane was on her parents' couch in Waltham, twenty-six-year-old Elle Montague was puttering around her brand-new home thirty miles away in woodsy Southborough. The TV was on low so her girls, five and three, didn't wake up, but Elle heard the news report nonetheless and felt a frisson of excitement. She quickly began weighing how much she and the family would have to sacrifice for her to take on such an intense commitment. It was a bit confusing that night as she processed how a civilian could spend so much time on an Army base and still be a civilian (she could), but she figured the details could be ironed out later.

They'd moved to the area for her husband Macon's consulting job and had found their church quick enough, but real friends were harder to come by for a stay-at-home mom. Elle would burst into any room with a smile and a hearty greeting for everyone; there was always a river of laughter bubbling beneath her words. But these New England women, they were tough. They had walls up and Elle was still so new here. This Army thing, whatever it was, would be something to do. It could be a way into her new life.

After two kids, Elle was ready to get back in fighting shape. She'd always had a naturally strong build, with a tight waist and solid muscle tone, so much so that shortly after she got engaged, a prominent law-enforcement agency took notice and began the process of recruiting her. But before she had a chance to prove herself, an agent took her aside and spoke frankly. *Choose,* they said. *Choose now between your fiancé and us. We've found that women can't be a wife and an agent.* Elle chose Macon without hesitation, and she didn't bother asking the obvious question: Did they tell male recruits the same thing about *their* fiancées? Of course they didn't.

She scribbled down the scientists' contact information and slept on it. Would Macon support something like this? How would babysitting work? How would they pay for it? She calculated the $500 they'd get at the end would cover much of it, but not all. By morning, Elle knew she was going for it, and she bounded out of bed with new purpose.

Nadine Nesbitt, who lived in the next town over, joined the study for very different reasons. The thirty-three-year-old mom of a young daughter was a successful insurance agent and was running hither and thither taking care of business while navigating an ongoing divorce. She heard about the experiment and thought, *I think I'll take on something else now.* Something huge to add to an already full life. Her first thought was, *How can I help prove that with proper training, women can do the jobs they want to do? I HAVE to do this.* Nadine wasn't someone who needed much sleep, which was a bonus, and she wasn't fearful of what the scientists might ask of her—she was champing at the bit.

Mary, Jane, Elle and Nadine were all accepted into the study early on in the recruiting process. But none of those hopeful young women could've known that a grenade was about to be lobbed into the scientists' carefully laid plans. Soon, I would learn why I wasn't hearing back about my application. Unbeknownst to me, I'd already been flatly rejected as a test subject. It might not matter, anyway, because the Pentagon was ready to cut the study loose.

It was the worst Valentine's Day surprise Everett and Pete had ever received. Their study had generated buzz in the Boston area, but then, suddenly, it went national—and not in a good way. The article splashed on the front page of the *Washington Times* on February 14, 1995, headlined "Why can't a woman be more like a man?", eviscerated the Natick study before it could start.

The conservative newspaper gave ample space for an outraged Retired Army Colonel Robert Maginnis to rail about the experiment's pointlessness. "The ludicrous notion that we can go out there and hire women and spend a phenomenal amount of time building them up to the equal of men just doesn't make any sense," Maginnis said. "We cannot afford social experiments with the military forces of this country."

Apparently no one told the good colonel he'd missed the point of the scientists' effort, which was to show that women could get strong *not* in a "phenomenal amount of time," but during the course of a normal day—before breakfast, on their lunch hours, after work. Also quoted in the piece was very concerned sociology professor Charles Moskos, whom I pictured wringing his hands on our behalf as he worried for our delicate frames: "In our haste to break the glass ceiling, let's hope we don't break women's bones." *Ouch!* I checked my own bones and found them in fine fettle; they didn't *seem* prone to shattering against any ceiling, glass, brass or otherwise.

Overdramatic as it was, the polemic made waves in Washington and beyond. It wasn't just a flash of bad PR—it was an excuse for detractors of women in combat to decry what they perceived as an attempt at an end run around the exclusion rule. It rattled Army brass, who had a low tolerance for controversy about women in its ranks and were already jittery, as tensions were rising over this issue even before the *Times* article. A month earlier, news stories emerged in which Georgia Republican Newt Gingrich, the newly installed Speaker of the House, was spouting off about women in the military. He reportedly told his class at Mind Extension University that women lacked the upper body strength to survive in combat and went on to describe the "infections" we constantly contract that make us unfit for service. Apparently, the man who ran for office on a family values ticket, who would divorce his first wife when she was being treated for cancer and cheat on his second wife with his third and then file for divorce shortly after she was diagnosed with Multiple Sclerosis, was all about protecting the female gender.

Gingrich was quoted as saying, "If upper-body strength matters, men win. They are both biologically stronger and they don't get pregnant. Pregnancy is a period of male domination in traditional society. On the other hand, if what matters is the speed by which you can move the laptop, women are at least as fast and in some ways better."

It was, of course, a woman who called Gingrich out on his crap. Days after reports of his comments emerged, during the inaugural session of the 104th Congress, Rep. Patricia Schroeder stood up on the house floor and took on the new speaker.

"I feel like I am taking the floor to defend men and women," Schroeder, a Democrat from Colorado, began. "[Gingrich] says, 'If combat means being in a ditch, then females have biological problems being in a ditch for thirty days because they get infections.' Well, I do not know of any medical status for this, and I would be very interested in having those facts..." Schroeder went on. "He says further,

'When it comes to men, men are like little piggies. You drop them in a ditch, and they will wallow and roll around in it.' Well, I am standing here defending my husband, my son, my uncles, my father. I mean, I have seen them in ditches, but they do not roll around like little piggies."

Gingrich had unwittingly expanded the talent roster for Ev's study. Stacey Coady, twenty-eight at the time and living in nearby Wellesley, went slack-jawed with disgust when she read his words. "I was following current events closely," she told me. "Newt Gingrich was saying we were inherently weaker than men. I took great offense." Around the same time, she saw the Natick scientists' call for volunteers. It was as if fate stood in front of her and handed her a way to clap back. "I was angry," Stacey explained. "And I knew that I was freakishly strong—I always had been."

Back at school in Bellingham, Mass., there was a group of boys who were routinely picked on, threatened and physically attacked. Stacey, who stands five-foot-ten and change, wasn't going to let it continue. "I used to walk kids, I didn't know they were gay at the time, but I used to walk those kids home so they wouldn't get beaten up. I knew I was strong enough, that I could disprove the premise that women were not strong enough to be in the military, because I knew I was stronger than your average guy."

It was, in fact, as if she'd been training her whole life for this moment. "I'm one of eight girls in my family," said Stacey, who applied and was quickly accepted into the study. "We were the Coady girls. We were on the fields playing every sport. When I was a kid in the seventies, because of Prop 2 ½ [an initiative to cap property taxes], they went to cut sports in our town—and they wanted to cut *girls* sports, but not boys. My father had us going around the neighborhood with flyers knocking on doors to get people not to permit this sexist decision. We did win in Bellingham. Those are the roots of my feminism. So I wasn't happy with Newt Gingrich."

The debate raged on in Washington after that, leading to the *Times* story about Everett and Pete's study. In it, Maginnis concluded that discriminating against women "is not about equal opportunity. It is about military readiness. Underline. Exclamation point. We cannot afford social experiments with the military forces of this country."

Turns out he was right about that second part. Our military has used female fighters to win wars since the American Revolution, when the famous "Molly Pitcher," who historians believe was actually Mary Ludwig Hays, took over from her wounded husband at the Battle of Monmouth and fired repeatedly as the British charged toward her. Years later, Deborah Sampson was shot while fighting as "Robert Shurtliff" for the Continental Army. To avoid being found out by medics who might catch a glimpse of her genitalia, she stole away and dug the bullet out of her own leg with a penknife and a sewing needle. Harriet Tubman is known for her heroic work on the Underground Railroad, but she was also a soldier and a spy. During the Combahee Ferry Raid in the Civil War, she charged in with an all-male unit and became the first woman in U.S. history to lead an armed military operation.

Much later, women ended up on the frontlines and were injured, killed and taken hostage in the Gulf War. After Desert Storm in 1991, Rep. Schroeder pointed out, "The Persian Gulf helped collapse the whole chivalrous notion that women could be kept out of danger in a war. We saw that the theater of operations had no strict combat zone, that Scud missiles were not gender-specific—they could hit both sexes and, unfortunately, did."

The issue, then, was not whether we should allow women in combat. They were already there. Women have *always* jumped into the fire, given their lives and experienced the same horrors of war as men. But due to the combat exclusion they *weren't equally recognized or compensated for their bravery*. However heroically and faithfully they served, they could never reap the full benefits and rewards bestowed on their male counterparts. Female fighters returned from war to be denied medals, awards, promotions and pay raises reserved only for those with an official record of serving on the frontlines. Military women continually slammed their heads on the so-called "brass ceiling" thanks to the combat ban.

Army Captain Linda Bray is a prime example of this unfair practice. During Operation Just Cause in 1989, Bray became the first woman in U.S. military history to lead a platoon into battle. As U.S. forces invaded Panama, she was given orders to neutralize the Panamanian Defense Force (PDF) canine unit and take out their communications. Under her command, the Military Police unit secured the kennel after a three-hour firefight—in other words, she and her team engaged in ground combat. But when Bray came home she was not granted the Combat Infantryman Badge. Instead, the Army gave her the Commendation Medal for Valor for meritorious achievement in a non-combat role because the rules said she never should've been in the fight at all. This blatantly discriminatory treatment spurred Pat Schroeder to once again jump in and stand up for women.

"First it was the academies, then the pilots, then combat…everything was like pushing a wheelbarrow up a hill with rubber handles. They were fighting all the way," Schroeder told me of her decades-long pursuit of equality for military women. "There was no reason they couldn't come up with the [physical fitness] standards and allow women [in combat roles]. The police and fire departments had already been doing it for years."

The Democratic representative known for her sharp wit and relentless advocacy first entered the Congress when Nixon was president and only fourteen women were members of the House. Schroeder's male colleagues welcomed her with a full script of sexist commentary, dubbing her "little Patsy" and loudly wondering why she wasn't home taking care of her kids. When a Congressman asked her point-blank how she could be a mother of two small children and a member of Congress at the same time, Schroeder shot back, "I have a brain and a uterus and I use both."

When she arrived on Capitol Hill she immediately set her sights on the big leagues, taking her place as the first female member of the conservative Armed Services Committee. Schroeder was watching closely in the aftermath of Linda Bray storming into battle. The captain's faultless performance didn't settle the controversy over women in combat; rather, it fired up the bitter debate anew. Even some feminists and progressives balked at her bravery, wary of any move that would send more women to the frontlines where they would kill and be killed like never before. Writer and pacifist Colman McCarthy wrote in a 1999 *Washington Post* piece that Bray's actions were nothing to celebrate: "War is a male ritual based on a hyper-masculine ethic that violence is rational. Linda Bray in Panama was less a victory for female rights than for male wrongs. She bought into traditional masculinism: Fists, guns, armies and killing are sensible solutions to problems."

Schroeder, who'd spoken out all over the media about Bray's heroics, wasn't apologizing. She proposed legislation to study the practicalities of letting women into all combat roles and did the media rounds with Bray to advocate for the new bill, and in doing so got pushback in places she never expected it. One visit to a prominent TV show was particularly ugly, Schroeder told me.

"The strangest thing was, I was doing a national morning show about this, and when I got done, the cameraman came out from behind the camera and started pounding on me," Schroeder said of the physical assault with disbelief still in her voice years later. "They immediately pulled him off. He just went *nuts* about women in combat. I wasn't really hurt, and people grabbed him and pulled him back. The head of the network's HR then called me and said this man had worked for them for years and was months away from having his pension vested, and they'd never seen this from him before. Should they let him go? I said 'No. I'm not going to be the one who keeps him from his pension.'

"It made me ponder all the things he had probably filmed all those years, and why nothing had gotten to him like women in combat, so much so that he would run the risk of losing his job. I can't understand it. To me it seems so fair."

Schroeder was met with resistance at every turn, including from top generals who kept their fists up on the issue of women in battle. "They had all this crap they came up with. It was like we were breaking into their tree house," she says. "No girls allowed. Here we were climbing up a tree and we were upsetting them. They made up all sorts of other stuff, including that we weren't strong enough."

She adds, "I remember one admiral testifying it would be OK to have women on ships, and afterward I said to him, 'wow, that's just wonderful, I remember last year you were opposed to them.' He said, 'I was, but my daughter has joined the D.C. police department and I realized she'd be safer on the ship.' And I thought, if we're going to have to do this one at a time it's going to take a long time. Thank goodness for daughters. I think they were a lot of the education process for these guys."

Schroeder's bill failed. Despite women fighting and dying for their country, the undervaluing of their contributions remained and the endless specious arguments for restricting women's opportunities remained in force: We'd freeze up under fire, ruin unit cohesiveness and threaten the safety of the infantry. We'd get pregnant or go wild with hormones. We lacked stamina. We'd cause men to sexually assault us.

"I heard every kind of idiot response you would ever believe from some generals saying men will be getting out of the tanks to open the doors for the women," Schroeder told me. "You just kind of shake your head and say, '*what?*'"

All this despite statistics showing women signing up to serve in all branches of the military were demonstrably better educated and posed less of a disciplinary problem than men, could fit into spaces male mechanics couldn't in order to fix planes and boats, and could gather life-saving intel from villages where female locals would never be permitted to speak to a strange man. Cutting out fifty percent of the population does nothing but harm the readiness of our armed forces. Women are, in short, essential. That said, we're also up against the unassailable fact that on average, men have more upper body strength than women (which was never a valid reason to keep us out of combat, especially with modern-day, far-removed "frontlines").

It seemed, then, that it was time to get to work closing that gap.

I was ready to stand up for military women. But there was radio silence from Everett and Pete, and I was extra freaked out because the Natick study was now officially a big story.

International headlines decried the study as an attempt to turn ladies into "Rambos" or "cyborgs," major TV networks, newspapers, and celebrity journalists including Jane Pauley were rumored to be circling, pressing for access to the scientists and the volunteers. Such naked exposure was out of the question for the DOD.

Andrea and I could only assume the scientists were mired in a sticky PR mess, for they were avoiding contact with us, but we had no idea just how tenuous the study's existence had become. Behind the scenes, all hell was breaking loose. The scientists fielded calls from their superiors at Fort Detrick in Maryland as soon as the offending edition of the *Washington Times* hit newsstands. Top brass recoiled at accusations they were trying to turn women into brutes, and even Everett's measured words in the interview he gave to the *Times* were like dangling flash paper over a bonfire for a newspaper with an agenda.

To the eager scientists' great dismay, the Pentagon ordered their strength study put on hold indefinitely. Instead of a March 13 start, Everett, Pete and their staff—including two top trainers—were left to sit on their hands and hope the political storm cleared. It was a terribly tense time for Everett and Pete. Not only did they have a team ready to train the women, but most volunteers had already been chosen. Some eighty civilian women from around Massachusetts had applied, a far greater number than the scientists had dreamed of attracting. Of those, they'd end up taking on forty-five, with number forty-six to be Marion Cavanaugh. But now, as media pressure mounted, the

DOD was left with a conundrum: They could let the study proceed and be plagued by a constant hum of publicity keeping it on front pages, or cancel it and create an even bigger story, maybe be accused of a cover-up, of backing down, of willfully leaving women behind. The scientists felt helpless as months of work seemed poised to go down the drain; Everett, as principal investigator, had everything to lose.

It seemed like all they could do was wait and continue working on other things.

And while they did, while things stayed unnervingly quiet, someone remembered me and my application letter. I didn't know it, but Everett and Pete had taken one look at my request for unfettered access and passed over me. But now, in these dire times, someone floated the idea that a cub reporter at the suburban newspaper down the road could be the solution to their problem. While details of the negotiation so many years on are hazy to those involved, I was told at the time that between the scientists and the public affairs office, a plan was hatched that was so crazy it just might work.

The idea was that if the Army let me—a small-town, pre-Internet reporter no one had heard of—sign on as a test subject, the national publicity would die down. It was brilliantly counterintuitive: Any journalist willing to endure the study for the full seven months would be allowed to cover it. The brass knew the more prominent the journalist, the less chance she'd be able or willing to take on something so time-intensive. And they were right. None of the others took the bait. When the call came giving the scientists the green light, it set a series of life-changing events in motion.

The national media pressure continued behind the scenes, but with the new plan in place, the uproar died down. Andrea arranged for the paper to buy me top-of-the line hiking boots and for our publisher—*not* the Army—to pay me the $500 the volunteers would get at the end of the study (old-school journalism would never permit accepting money from those we cover). But first, Andrea set firm boundaries: My articles would not be vetted by Army public affairs, nor could they dictate what I could write about our experience.

The day I found out she struck a deal was the day I realized how much I wanted to be a part of it. Trying my hiking boots on, feeling the stiff uppers supporting my ankles like little fortresses, *that* was the moment it got real. Yet I still didn't ask myself the hard questions dangling in front of my face. It would be years before I stepped back and considered the obvious: Why would a woman *want* to be in combat, anyway? Why was I so determined to do something—even if it was a mere ripple in the tide of change—that could send more women into harm's way, and possibly to their deaths? That didn't concern me, not at that time. I was ready to jump in and get my hands dirty, and Everett told me there was just one more box to tick: I had to pass the Army's physical.

I sat on a table in my flimsy paper gown while an Army doctor examined me. I was twenty-four, a regular exerciser, non-smoker and former athlete who kept active. I'd been told that showing up on the base in "average shape" was just dandy. I wasn't worried about passing this first test as the sandy haired man probed and prodded me, listened to my heart, took my blood pressure. This doctor silently made notes on his clipboard. Then he looked up at me.

"I can't clear you."

He said it as if discussing the weather: *My, it's unseasonably cold today.*

"*What*?" How could a man decide I wasn't fit for this in five minutes? "Why?"

"You have high blood pressure." He shrugged; that was that.

"That's ridiculous. I'm twenty-four years old."

He offered no recommendations or remedy, no chance to breathe and see if I could relax a bit and maybe rule out white-coat syndrome. He didn't say, *There's medication we could try. Let's see what we can do. Your numbers aren't* that *high.*

"We can take another reading," he finally said, perhaps because my face reflected the spectrum of humiliation, fear and panic I was feeling. I didn't bother asking what the numbers were. It didn't matter to me then; this was a pass/fail situation. I breathed, he squeezed. I closed my eyes, willed my body to calm down, to slow the pumping, to beat the damn cuff. With one final, crackling rip of the Velcro, my chances died.

"Three readings. All high. There's nothing I can do."

"I feel fine, though. Can't I do the study anyway? Keep an eye on the pressure? I've never had this problem before." No one had ever flagged my blood pressure.

"No way," the doctor replied. "Absolutely not. Sorry."

He made it clear it wouldn't help for me to speak to the scientists and beg for an override or an exception. That's what the doctor was here for; his *one job* was to screen out danger, liability, and the predictable potential for sudden death. Heavy weights are kryptonite for people with high blood pressure. And we now know that yo-yo dieters are at a higher risk for heart attack and strokes.

As the doctor uttered the final verdict, I felt defeated. I was stuck in a spiral of hunger, overeating and a complete loss of control; there's nowhere to go but up from 800 calories a day, and anything I was taking in beyond that was being stored as fat. That condition was paired with an infinite hunger no food could satisfy. I didn't know then about the Minnesota Starvation Experiment, a World War II-era study that put thirty-six men through six months of semi-starvation. On 1,570 calories a day, some subjects reported a descent into madness, food obsessions, nightmares, and bottomless hunger that was never satiated once the calorie restrictions were removed. I didn't need to be skinny; I wanted to be healthier, lighter, and more comfortable in my jeans. I didn't see a way out without extreme exercise.

Now it looked like that would be taken away. I wasn't sure how much fight I had left to push my way into the Army's world, and thought perhaps all the obstacles were a sign. This latest turn of events was my own fault, and I berated myself in the harshest terms with words I wouldn't speak to my worst enemy. I was too embarrassed to talk to my editors about it. At home, that night, I thought about what a moment means.

About how one minute, one second, one day can define a life, and can set you on a course to your true north. I thought about how I'd been bullied throughout my childhood and about what it means to be strong. I thought, I have a choice. I can stand strong and face the shame I felt after the doctor's appointment. I could confront it and push it away. I *would* fight, I decided, for the ten-year-old me standing on that playground with a ring of boys laughing and calling me horrible names. *That* is the girl who would kick ass in the Army. She would take these bones, that muscle, and yes, even the fat, and make it work as the machine it was made to be. *That* girl would make *this* body soar.

I waited until my roommate left for work one morning and called Everett in the quiet. Busy as he was with his own problems, he listened to me. He is not someone who pretends to hear you or engages in active listening; there are no *uh-huh, uh-huh, mm hmms* to interrupt your sharing. Ever thoughtful and decisive, he heard me, and then he said... *Yes.* One word and it was done. He offered to let me to sign some sort of waiver, and then I would be able to join his study. Everett showed no stress or judgment during that discussion, only understanding—but more than that, he showed an investment in me. It was a poignant revelation after the doctor's blithe dismissal. The scientists wanted me. They *really* wanted me.

Would I drop dead mid-bench press? Keel over with a cardiac event on the backpack hike? Who knew. But the scientists clearly felt I had a good chance of surviving their regimen, and they signed off. I was, once and for all, *in.*

3

More than you can chew

Ev, Pete and their two hand-picked trainers—Eric Lammi, forty, and Chris Palmer, twenty-five—stood at the front of a large conference room on the Natick base and surveyed the motley crew before them. The four men who would lead the study saw women who were quiet, fidgety, a bit awkward, impatient, shy, nervous. The dozens of potential subjects in that room were everything at once, but most of all they were out of their element. They were casually dressed civilians invading a regimented world whose inhabitants were conducting the serious business of defending our country. The women wore baggy shorts and raggedy T-shirts, college sweatshirts and messy ponytails in a land of pressed uniforms, perfect posture and hair shorn to strict Army standards.

This would be one of the few times all the subjects would be in the same room together. Based on the times they'd indicated they could work out every day, they'd be broken out into four small groups for the duration: A-Group would train before work, B at mid-morning, C at mid-afternoon, and D after work.

Everyone should have known by then what they were signing up for, but Eric wanted there to be no mistake about how hard the next seven months would be. "This is not gonna be sitting on a stationary bike reading *People* magazine," he told the group. "You're all going to be athletes at the end of this—and it'll be one of the hardest things you'll ever do."

Nadine, the insurance agent with an attachment to the color purple, didn't need a pep talk. "Come on—let's do this!" She shouted from the audience. "What are we waiting for?"

Not everyone was so eager. A few people appeared shaky, even scared. Study volunteer Denise LePage noted the trepidation among some potential subjects upon hearing the team's harsh honesty about what lay ahead. The guys told them how important a full commitment was, how hard it could get, and informed the group they could miss ten sessions in all—any more than that and they'd be dismissed from the experiment. Denise sat among them, watched the wavering ones, and shook her head. She had no intention of letting this opportunity pass her by. She was a landscaper at the time, and planned to slot the training into her work schedule whatever it took. As she watched a few people file out before the meeting was over, she shook her head and remarked to another subject, "Look at them *adiosing*. I guess they're afraid of actual work."

Later that day, the team—Eric, Everett, Pete and Chris—dissected how it all went, and wondered who among the group would make the final decision to show up when the study started. "It was a very eclectic group that we saw in front of us," Eric observed. "We saw women who appeared like they hadn't been working out all that much, and then others who looked like they had. We had various body types, heights, sizes, shapes. Everybody had their own reasons for joining the study. Some people wanted to get in shape. Others wanted to participate in something that was big and was going to help female soldiers."

That first orientation wasn't a long one, and Nadine would soon get her wish to get started, because the next order of business was to put us all to the test for two straight weeks.

On the first day of the study, as the trees around Lake Cochituate began their early May explosion, forty-five civilian women swarmed the Army base on a promise. They came on motorcycles, in minivans, on bicycles, in sports cars and on foot. They left children with sitters, sacrificed sleep, left parents shaking heads at this bonkers undertaking, and paused their lives to do one special thing that would certainly cost them, but perhaps pay them in a multitude of ways, too.

I drove my sporty red 1988 Toyota Celica with one pink door toward the base entrance. I stopped at the guard's shack, an intimidating checkpoint that put me on edge. A guard approached my window, and I noted the name embroidered on his camouflage jacket: *O'HARA*.

"I.D. please."

"Yes, *Sir*!" I almost saluted the frowning young man out of sheer nerves, but thankfully stopped myself; I didn't know the rules here, and I wanted to avoid insulting a soldier on my first day.

I handed him my license and he checked his list. "Drive straight ahead until you see the lake," he said, handing it back, squinting and pointing. I decided this O'Hara guy didn't like me. "The lot where you're allowed to park is right there, and the training building will be on your right. You can't miss it."

Wrong, O'Hara. *I* could miss it. I'd been cursed at birth with a horrendous sense of direction, and to make things worse every building I passed looked the same—square, dark, industrial. Thanks to O'Hara's directions, I spotted the lot up ahead on the edge of the lake. One minute into this journey and I felt like a fraud. I drove past uniformed and camo-clad men and women, and I thought about how these people signed up knowing the might risk their lives and so many pried bravery from deep within their fear to protect my comfortable life. Did I have any right to be afraid today?

The base appeared as functional and basic as you'd expect. Full of hard lines with everything in its place, the installation was dotted with drab, flat-roofed buildings and the occasional random tarp covering a mystery lump. Still, as I parked in our designated parking area at the outer edge, I could see it would be a lovely place to pass three seasons. The property was set on the edge of Lake Cochituate with thick, full woods that would burst into blazing color come autumn.

I turned off the car, gathered the courage to go inside, and remembered why I'd fought to be here. Too many people in power didn't want it to happen. Too many thought we would fail. Military women needed us to do this, and do it well. Another of Maginnis's snappy quotes ran through my mind: *I don't care how long you exercise this group of women up in Massachusetts. You will never bring them up to a point where if men went through the same experiment, the women would ever be equal.*

I stepped out, slammed my car's lone pink door shut, walked toward the training room that would become like home to me, and thought, *Well, Colonel, I'm about to meet some women up in Massachusetts who are going to prove you wrong.*

All along I'd been picturing my fellow volunteers as Glamazons. I was ready to walk in and see *Rocky IV*-era Bridgette Nielsen spotting track star FloJo on the bench press while volleyball goddess Gabrielle Reece jumped rope next to them. I'd always adored women, taken to them, held my girlfriends as close as kin, because they were; we were each other's temporary family until it was time to launch into our real lives. Women are the strong ones. The smart ones. The intuitive ones. I walked toward that open door, the gaping maw that would suck me into a new life and hold me there until it was ready to spit me out, and I was almost more worried about impressing the women than the scientists and trainers. I was expected to write killer front-page features about our journey, and I needed my comrades to trust me off the bat.

I stood outside for a moment in my lightweight, roomy tracksuit pants and loose T-shirt, then pulled the door open. I strode in, blinking to adjust out of the sunlight. The place was bustling with scientists and trainers and volunteers, their voices echoing in the converted Army warehouse that smelled faintly of sweaty socks and mechanic's grease. With high ceilings and industrial lighting, the design motif of our workout room was unabashedly utilitarian and packed with weight machines, contraptions, steel boxes galore, and, ominously, sand bags.

Everett greeted me fleetingly as he prepared for our session. I grew more anxious, as if endless shots of espresso were being pushed into my veins. My alleged high blood pressure was possibly spiking, but I'd never tell. The other women were unsmiling or fidgeting nervously. Our leaders were too busy to make introductions. I waved across the room to my newspaper's staff photographer Ken McGagh, who'd been assigned to follow us with his camera for the study's duration, then turned to the door as a woman bounded in. She made her entrance with a grand smile, waving and calling out hellos that were somehow both shy and unabashedly loud at the same time. She was five-foot-five with wavy chestnut hair falling just below her ears and was dressed in a basic cream T-shirt and mom-jeans shorts.

"Hi! I'm Elle. Oh my gosh. Isn't this *wild*?" She giggled as she took a good look around.

Those of us in the vicinity agreed it was wild, and I felt the scattered group start to relax for a moment. We checked each other out. There were about twenty of us in this space, and as it turned out, *I* was the closest to Brigitte Nielsen by virtue of being giant and blonde. We were regular people with regular-women bones and teeth and body shapes. It was designed that way. The rules of human subject research dictated that Ev and his team could not single out certain people and say, *You look like you have potential—we're gonna take you.* Once the investigators establish the criteria—in this case falling into the right age range and being in good health—they're not supposed to pick and choose who they think will succeed, because that would bias the study.

I noted our fashion choices were equally standard: There wasn't a tight tank-top or designer outfit to be seen. Less than half of the forty-six test subjects seemed to be in attendance. I scanned the room and thought about whether this was a group that could change history or not, and then Everett signaled it was time to start. There were no formalities, no welcome ceremony, neither pomp nor circumstance. "Today will be fairly easy," he informed us. "Just some body assessments and things of that nature."

Body assessments. I felt like telling them there was no need. I'd assessed my own body and found it wanting. They split us up into groups, and I was led away along with Elle and a few others upstairs to a small room with a treadmill and machinery outfitted with an ominous-looking tube and a some sort of mask.

"Who's first?" asked a man waiting there.

"Do *what?*" Elle, wide-eyed, said under her breath.

I shot her a look of solidarity. "Fuck that," I agreed, not so much under my breath as I should have. The man then explained to us we were about to embark on a test of our maximum aerobic ability which would, as the attendant put it, "require running until close to exhaustion."

"I'll go." Elle stepped up despite her obvious reservations, and as she did, she announced, "I can't even run a mile! I've had two kids and I haven't worked out in forever."

The man strapped the mask to her mouth and clipped a glorified clothespin to her nose. I felt claustrophobic just looking at her. When the guy started up the belt, I saw panic in Elle's eyes. Sweat was soon running down her face, and she turned a ghostly grey as she ran faster on a steeper incline. The man pushed more buttons. The hill got steeper still. He pushed again, and the belt sped up. The only sounds were the whir of the machine, the thumping of her feet on the belt, and the Darth Vader noises from the mouthpiece. Elle ran until the man chose to slow things down and take her out of her misery. I was closest to the machine, and I felt a clear expectation I would go next. And then, unbidden, two words slipped out of my mouth.

"I can't."

No one seemed to hear except for Elle, standing in front of me with her chest heaving and tendrils of damp hair falling around her face.

"Yes, you can."

I sensed that the girl in the jeans shorts was going to stare me down until I stepped up, so I did, and I realized with a start this could be the easiest run I'd ever do.

Stopping mid-song wasn't an option, and more to the point, there would *be* no song apart from the beat of my own feet. The man strapped the mask to my face, and I thought, *This will be OK*, and then he clipped my nostrils shut. I had one choice if I was going to get through this: Breathe and put one foot in front of the other. I did. Until I felt sick, until I thought I couldn't go any faster, until the man decided I'd absorbed all the O2 by body would allow that day and stopped the belt. When I finished my turn, I had to know how I stacked up.

"Did I do OK?" I asked through huffing and puffing.

He replied, "Next!"

That was bad, but I knew worse was to come, like the trailer pull I'd heard so much about. This was not a fear shared by another test subject called Jean Heafey. She decided that day that no test would be worse than the VO2 max. When she alighted on the belt, she donned the mask, started running, and quickly grew inwardly enraged. The twenty-three-year old Toys 'R' Us employee had always been athletic and had a savage competitive streak, but *this* pissed her off. The lack of control. The pain. The nose clip. Jean wanted off, and her thoughts grew ever more frantic as she ran. *It's hard to breathe. What is this? It's too claustrophobic. Frick it, I'm just going to end it right now. Screw you guys! You don't want to tell me how long I'm going to run? I'm going to stop.* But of course she never did, not until the man halted the ride on his own terms.

I was led to another room for a DEXA (short for dual energy X-ray absorptiometry) scan. I lay on my back in a machine that reminded me of a tanning bed, but instead of bronzing my skin, it measured every teaspoon of blubber on my body, every ounce of muscle, every sliver of bone. The DEXA was oddly relaxing. But again, not for Jean. She is the only test subject I ever spoke to who named this test as one of her worsts. "You had to lie still for like forty-five minutes," she grumbled afterward. "For me, that in itself was a challenge."

What was up with this Jean person? Sitting still was one of my favorite pastimes. Didn't she know the bad things were yet to come—the trailer pull, the backpack, the timed squats? Not to mention the innocuously named "skin-fold" test, which was an irredeemable insult. Back in the training room, Everett beckoned me over with cold metal forceps and proceeded to tug at all the fattest places on my body, the ones I despised most, and measure them to calculate my body fat percentage. *Lift your arm.* Pinch. *Good; now I'll get your back fat.* Pinch. *Don't move. Good.*

They saved the worst for last. When I was led over to the final machine, I recoiled and tried to think of a way out. I thought about making a run for it. There it stood, pure existential evil, waiting to torment me: The Scale of Doom. I knew I'd gained weight, because my clothes were tightening daily like a slow-motion Incredible Hulk, but I feared learning the actual number would send me to the nearest Donut Depot before you could say Boston cream. I estimated I'd put on maybe twenty-five or thirty pounds out of the sixty I'd lost on the starvation diet. That estimate was based on wishful thinking and eyeballing myself in the mirror while sucking in.

I heard a loud, sharp groan mixed with a rueful little laugh from a woman who had just stepped on. "Oh *maaannn*," the woman cried. It was Elle, giggling again. She put her hand over her mouth, then went on, "Aw, *man*! One-thirty-eight? Are you *kidding* me? OK—I've got to drop eight. Eight pounds. I gotta get to one-thirty and then we'll see."

Pete was marking her weight down. I was way worse off than Ms. Eight Fricking Pounds. I'd *kill* for one-thirty-anything. I side-eyed her and wondered how anyone could be that happy all the time.

Pete flicked his eyes in my direction. "Hop on."

I got a grip and stepped up. Pete moved the dreaded balance, *tap, tap, tap*. When he finally stopped, I opened one eye. It wasn't pretty. I'd never sought to cross the border out of the one-hundreds. I *loved* the one-hundreds, but now these scientists had forced me to leave for an extended stay in two-hundred-land. Still, even as I wallowed in my hyperbolic horror in the face of this inanimate piece of machinery, I was aware none of this really mattered, and that perspective is badly needed in these situations. Look to your right and there is someone you are dying to be; look to your left and there is someone who would kill to be you. Problem was, I'd fought for years not to drive myself crazy trying to match anyone else's image of what I should look like, but I *did* want to feel fit and comfortable in my own skin. Right then, I didn't. I stepped off the scale and finally it was over. I was told to come back the next day for more. More of what, they didn't say.

I rolled back my Celica's sunroof and raced back to my basic apartment with its standard white slat blinds, grey carpet, eggshell walls and poster of a pouting, ponytailed *Legends of the Fall*-era Brad Pitt on my closet wall. It was three-thirty. I had no idea how I was going to clean up, get back to the office, and concoct a news story or two before end of business. I checked the answering machine while stripping off.

Beeeeep.

"Hey, it's me…" Began a male voice.

We're already at "it's ME?" Please stop.

"…I, uh, haven't heard from you, so wanted to make sure we're on for tomorrow night…give me a call."

Why are you being so horrible? Don't crowd me.

Beeeep.

The voice belonged to Ford Simmons, a guy around my age I'd met when I was working on a story about a local charity. He had a vague job in "sales and marketing" and was volunteering his time to help the charity increase donations. We'd embarked on an innocent fling, but lately he'd been scaring me shitless because I suspected he genuinely liked me.

Meanwhile, in the shower after my first session, I tried to forget I'd gained twenty pounds in one day. Denial, I felt, was often the best way to handle difficult things. I thought about whether to blow Ford off or keep chugging along until something better came along—for me *or* him. I preferred torrid affairs when I could find them, but it had been awhile since I was bombarded with offers. It's a funny thing, isn't it? The thinner you are, the more men want to be around you. The fatter you are, the more invisible you become, which for some of us can be a welcome respite from the pressing horniness of the American male. In any case, I was more interested in fun than longevity just then. I never believed in one soul mate. My idea of the perfect partner was a person you could stand for long periods of time, who pulls the plug on the claustrophobia, who knocks down the walls, opens up the plains, and tells you to run, run, run as far as you can, and then you can go back when you're ready, safe and free at the same time. All clues pointed to my never finding anything close to that, but I intended on having a good time along the way.

Catherine: 2013

Catherine Afton walked out of her local Army recruitment office and knew it wasn't the career for her. Her father saw the mismatch just as clearly.

"Let's go home," he suggested. "Maybe this wasn't such a good idea."

"We have other places to try," Catherine, a high-school track star who also excelled at academics, replied. "The Marine Corps office isn't far."

It was the winter of 2013, and the seventeen-year-old high school senior's life was largely devoted to college applications. She had the grades and the ambition to offer the best schools, but she didn't have a way to pay for the elite institutions she planned to apply to. Her dream college was one of the top universities in the country and even if she got in, Catherine would have to find the money to pay for it. She drew charts. She made lists. She did her research, but all the calculations in the world couldn't conjure cash out of thin air.

That was when her father had a light-bulb moment. It was a bit out of left field perhaps, especially for a family with no military experience to speak of, but a last-ditch strategy was called for, so off they'd marched to the recruitment offices. But now, as she prepared to enter the Marines' den, Catherine reconsidered.

Maybe I'm not good enough for such an elite school, she thought. *Maybe it's better to be a medium fish in a medium pond.*

She couldn't picture what life would be like in the military, nor grasp what it would look like to be a soldier. "I didn't understand there was a difference between [the Marines and the Army]. I didn't understand what the military was," she admitted later.

Still, it wasn't Catherine's style to give up. She and her father walked into the Marine Corps recruiting office, at once intimidating and enticing with its aura of adventure, danger and the unknown, and announced themselves. The laser-focused recruiters quickly sensed a star in their midst. (Side note: Catherine was very uncomfortable with my interest in her story—"there are so many others, I'm not special"—and, like other military women I spoke to, never sought to be singled out. Despite her discomfort, she graciously agreed to speak with me because of how the Natick strength study directly affected her life.)

"We went in," Catherine recalls, "and they were very

good at convincing me the Marine Corps was perfect for me. I took a short academic test. They got my results and said, 'you have to apply for the officer program. Look into ROTC to pay for school—you have to be an officer afterward.' I left that day with paperwork in hand."

The high-school senior went home and took stock. She scanned her charts and lists and took a hard look at the numbers, and the military was suddenly looking quite good. "I went to a different office next. They showed me a video and I ran the physical fitness test. They said I ran faster than all the guys before me," Catherine remembers. "I went home and thought about it. They talked about leadership opportunities, and even though I was captain of sports teams in high school, I didn't really know what it meant to be a leader. They said the Marines were the toughest, and I liked that; I wanted to go the furthest."

The Reserve Officer Training Corps (ROTC), a program ensconced at some 1,700 campuses across the country, pays for college and gives students a guaranteed career after graduation. With her grades, SAT scores and physical fitness level, Catherine got into her dream school and qualified for ROTC easily. Her lists had led to a pot of gold: college would be paid for. The road was rising to meet Catherine Afton.

May 1995

On that first day of testing I managed to get back to the office before five, leaving about two hours to craft a story for the next day's paper. No one in the busy newsroom asked me how my Army experience went. They had a paper to put out.

After I sent my story to my editor, I turned my attention back to the Army. I started two separate diaries: One in a fresh reporter's notebook that would serve as a guide for my upcoming articles, and another in a sky-blue journal I expected would live buried in my closet for decades to come. Before I left the office, knowing Ford would still be at work, I left a message on his home machine cancelling tomorrow's date. I'd be too tired from the Army and work, I told him. I'd see him around.

The next day at the base, I formally met our trainer for the first time. Eric Lammi, all six-foot-three of him, stood in shadow in our training room, which was once again humming with the quiet energy of psyched-up people who didn't know each other yet. Eric was forty years old, lean, tanned, and in possession of a full pate of golden blond hair. At that moment he was focused on a hunk of pine furniture resembling a high-school shop class project. Unvarnished and entirely random in the otherwise metal-heavy area of the great room, the unit had two shelves: one at thirty inches and one at sixty inches.

I approached him. "Eric, right?"

"I'm your trainer," he replied. He had a piercing voice and a Boston accent, so the third word came out somewhere between *trainar* and *trainah.*

"Then who's that?" I pointed to a young guy I'd noticed yesterday.

"Chris Palmer. The other trainer."

"Thanks. That's helpful."

Eric offered a twinkly-eyed eyebrow raise at my insolence. I checked Chris out from a distance. At twenty-five, he was prettier, younger, and more muscular than Eric. There was another key difference between them: Chris wore a wedding ring on his left hand. Eric didn't.

"OK, everyone." Everett called out. "Circle up for box lifts."

We dutifully gathered around the shelving unit. Everything was unfamiliar to me, making those initial moments feel chaotic and unsettling. We formed a crescent as Eric introduced us to the metal boxes we'd get to know better than our own mothers. They were a dark, icy grey, scratched up with sharp corners and iron handles.

Eric demonstrated how we should simulate vital military tasks in which soldiers must lift heavy equipment and supplies. We'd be taking boxes from the floor to table height (thirty inches) and from table height to a high shelf (sixty inches), and we were told proper technique must include "maintenance of a smooth lifting motion, left-right body symmetry, an arched back, and use of the legs in preference to the back."

I stepped up to the makeshift shelf. Eric loaded a round weight plate into my box, and as I crouched and grabbed the handles, I thought, *They're all looking at my butt, aren't they?* I felt my pants strain against my rear end as I took hold of the cold metal. The group had gone quiet. *Yep. They're looking at my butt.* I wanted to run, but instead I straightened up and brought the box easily to 30 inches. And then it was someone else's turn to be the center of attention, and she did her job quickly and quietly.

This test was progressive, so we went in rounds to give each subject a rest between attempts. The next woman appeared more nervous than I was, even as she set the metal on the shelf with a satisfying *thud.* On my next turn Eric added another weight. I was still acutely aware of the group behind me, but also of a building tide of excitement racing through the room. The boxes were cold and dead, the subjects jittery and energized, and I was there in the middle, trying to ignore it all and lift the next box with what I thought was good form. On my next turn Eric added yet more weight. This one was *not* doable. I lifted it to my waist, but struggled to bring it up to the shelf. I was going to drop it; I was going to fail on day two. I thought about the woman doing this as a job. Would she drop the box? Would a female soldier loading supplies next to a man *stop*? What would she do?

I grunted, "Can I use my thighs to rest it on? Or—" I managed to get it up a bit higher—"my elbows?"

"You can use any body part and any means of getting the box to the shelf," one of the guys replied. It was digging into my leg, and then the handle rested on my wrist, and somehow my elbow got involved. It hurt—a lot.

I wasn't going to make it. A few attempts into it and I was, without warning, toast. But....wait. I *wasn't.* In one flash, one blip in time, I was saved. I don't know who started it, but in a beautiful millisecond, the women around me erupted. I felt it before I heard it. There was a *Woo!,* then a *Come on, girl, you can DO it!* , and there were cheers and claps. I wriggled that box up; I lifted that thing like a car that had fallen on a child, embracing my grunts and funny faces, using my thighs, my waist, my breasts, each a stopping point to gain leverage. So much for "proper technique."

When it was my turn again Eric filled my box with more weight, and the women filled my soul with more power. Up the box went. The next one after that…well, that thing wasn't going to budge past my knees no matter what I did, but by then the tone of the room had changed, the next woman was ready, and I was there for her. *You. Can. Do. It.* Those words stayed with me. Even when the goal seems impossible, even when too many people say you can't, tell yourself these words: *I can do it.*

Elle lifted the most that day and gave us a lesson in genetics. It didn't matter that she hadn't worked out in forever and was never a serious athlete, that she was older than I was and smaller in stature. We were all blown away, but Elle only tilted her head and smiled. "I carry the kids everywhere," she would shrug. "It makes me strong."

I thought it was a ridiculous assertion. If having kids made you excessively fit, we could put all the moms in the special forces and be done with it. But I couldn't argue back, because the fact remained that Elle was stronger than all of us in C-Group, whatever the reason.

As Mary from A-Group put it, the progressive box lift was a special kind of tough. It didn't last long, but it was frustrating. You could lift it or you couldn't—that was that.

"There were some things that just beat me," Mary told me in one of my interviews with her. "The ones where you needed pure strength like the progressive box lift—I sucked at those. It didn't matter how hard I tried on the final lift. I couldn't do it."

Like all of us, she gave everything to go harder, faster and stronger, but sometimes it didn't feel like enough.

The next day, at the base checkpoint, I tried to charm O'Hara with a cheery yet respectful hello. I got a curt wave to drive on. If I didn't know better, I'd say he didn't want us messy, undisciplined civilians traipsing around his base. I parked by the lake and headed to the training room. When I walked in, I found it eerily quiet. The hustle and bustle was gone, and its place stood five quiet souls waiting for direction. Soon there were six, as I turned to greet another woman walking in.

And then Eric focused on us. "Welcome to C-Group," he said, but I heard "Welcome to Thunderdome." The seven of us who'd been led willingly into this cage together glanced around at each other. Everett appeared from behind the cubicles against the wall, and the team led us to a contraption in the back corner that looked like a half-baked, oversized mousetrap game. The homemade conveyor system was staffed by two grad-school assistants—interns who would assist with our study for the coming months—wearing ear muffs, and we stood in front of it making silent eye contact and waiting for instructions. I was covertly sizing up the other subjects: Who would be the best? Who would struggle, maybe give up? Who would drag us down? The answer to all questions right now was, *Maybe me.*

Everett stood over a box. "Pick it up, then walk as fast as you can to the other end of the line"—he pointed to a spot about twenty feet away—"and set it on the belt. It will then roll back around to where our assistants are standing to push it to you again." The interns smiled and waved at us like we were about to board an exciting amusement-park ride. "Do *not* run with the box," Ev instructed as he ran back to pick up another. "You should, however, sprint as fast as you want on the way back. The object is to load as many boxes as you can in ten minutes."

We learned each box weighed forty pounds, the shelf was fifty-two inches high, and we'd carry the boxes twenty-five feet.

"Looks fun," Elle joked after Everett's demo.

"We'll start with you," Eric said to her.

Elle donned her earmuffs, Eric hit his timer, and the clanging and slamming began. Elle jogged over to the shelf carrying a box the size of a standard microwave oven. I quickly learned why the noise protectors were necessary—the sound of metal boxes pounding and scraping against the conveyor belt saturated the great room with a deafening cacophony. After a few minutes of picking up boxes and putting them down again, Elle began to slow, her chest heaving as she tried to catch her breath.

"You can do it, Elle!" someone shouted. "Keep going. You're almost there."

Everyone was clapping now. Elle picked up her pace

again. "Come on, keep going!" I yelled, knowing there was every chance she couldn't hear me. "You've got this!"

When Eric called time, Elle threw down her box and, heaving so badly I thought she might pass out, breezed by us all to walk it off. I would find out later she had asthma, yet I never heard her complain about her struggles to breathe.

"Sara. You're up." Eric shot a look at me.

I stepped up and grabbed the handles. On *Go!,* I went, and I found an odd sort of satisfaction in the rhythm of it. The forty pounds wasn't much, and because I was five-nine it wasn't tough to get the box up to the shelf. But then, out of nowhere, I burned out. Every muscle felt like it was seizing up, my lungs were at capacity, and I felt woozy. I stopped and bent over, trying to catch my breath. "Do. Not. Stop." Eric ordered. "Even if you slow down to a crawl, *keep moving.* Pace yourself."

Pace yourself. I was not a pacer. I'm not wired for moderation; it has always been all or nothing with me. I am about the peaks and valleys, and right then I was deep in the latter. I pushed through and upped my speed because I could feel a room full of eyes on me. When Eric called time, I let out an involuntary scream. I set the box on the ledge, tried to catch my breath, and only then noticed everyone was cheering for me.

"Amazing! You *owned* those boxes," Elle said, and slapped me hard on the back.

I let myself be proud. I *had* owned those boxes—and I hadn't given up even as the pain spread through me and challenged me to quit. The rest of the women took their turns, each one giving her last spark of energy. Nadine was the lithe, speedy runner, but wasn't so comfortable with this clunky, repetitive weight. Others who weren't so tall found the high shelf a hindrance. Marion, the study's one soldier, treated it like a job. I watched hundreds of metal boxes move by the sheer power of women, and I felt the first hint that these empty squares would become everything: a symbol of the things I couldn't do, the things I'd failed at in my life so far, what I feared and what I loved, the hurdles I'd cleared and those I'd had to find a way around.

The following day, the seven sore women of C-Group watched Everett demonstrate a new and exciting twist on the box lift. This time, we wouldn't be running—this was the box lift *minus* the carry. As the first woman got going, I shot a look to Marion, wearing a grey T-shirt with "ARMY" emblazoned across the chest, her thick auburn hair in a low bun.

"So what you're saying is, Army people have to lift a shitload of boxes," I said to her as we watched Everett.

She kept her eyes on the boxes.

"I'm Sara," I said. "The reporter covering the study."

"I know." She watched the curly-haired Amanda crouching.

"You lift a lot of boxes in your line of work?"

Clang. Grunt. Thump.

"Yes," the soldier gave in. "Into the backs of trucks, out of the backs of trucks, onto storage room shelves. We lift a lot of boxes."

"Sara!" Eric nodded to me. I stepped up and grabbed the box handles as he started his timer with one thumb and a sharp command: *Ready, set, go!* It took about a minute before my lungs felt ready to explode. I had assumed this test would be the easier one because of the no running, but I was tragically wrong. That twenty-five-foot jog had been a rest. *This* had no breather, and ten minutes felt like an hour.

When it was over, I shook out my hands and massaged my palm and its fleshy base. "Anyone else have numb thumbs?"

"It's the handles," Everett said helpfully.

"Definitely the handles," I agreed.

"Check this out," one woman said, rolling up her T-shirt sleeve to show us a row of purple bruises along her underarm.

"I can beat that." I raised one pant leg. There were splotches the size of golf balls and one that looked like a ragged scoop of blackberry ice cream, purple, blue and new. I have photos of that time, and the sheer number of contusions on display is alarming, but also a brand of bravery, I thought. A mark of spirit.

That night, I went home to a quiet apartment and crashed out on the couch with a glass of Roommate's pink Crystal Lite. After a long shower, I added water to the Pitcher That Shall Not Be Touched so Roommate wouldn't know of my thievery, then dragged myself out to the Town Hall for a seven p.m. meeting about the sewers or the school budget or mowing on the Town Green, I can't remember exactly what the big issue was. I raced back to the newsroom and wrote two stories about what happened and why any of it mattered to the people who lived in the town.

On my way home after midnight, I braced for another voicemail from Ford. I'd have to deal with him sooner rather than later. Just because I was in/around the Army now didn't mean I could avoid other aspects of my life.

You have no new messages, the smug robot voice told me when I got home. *Good. Great!*

Ford wasn't the only friend I hadn't talked to in the past ten days. Even before testing was completed, I found the study to be all-consuming, and I'd already started to let everything and everyone else fall by the wayside.

As much as the box tests raised my hopes of my ability to help the cause of women's strength, the next task ground them under one sharp stiletto. We were led to a patch of the training room where two glorified measuring sticks awaited us: One stuck to the floor, the other standing vertical.

"Jump," Eric said to me as my toe edged toward the line.

"How high?" I replied.

"You're going to be trouble," he said.

I would be. I was going to be trouble for all of these people, and not just in the *Ha ha* way he meant. First was the standing long jump, and as I crouched low I begged gravity to let me go, but alas, as I rose up and tried to pull my feet off the ground, I felt like a rhinoceros doing ballet. "We'll work on that," Eric said into his clipboard after a few tries.

I watched the others go. Nadine approached the line with a furrowed brow and made *one-hundred-percent sure* her toes were behind the line. Marion stepped forward and got on with it. Elle snapped to attention like a coiled spring. Amanda was an affable, bespectacled woman of about thirty. She walked in with oversized lenses and Bermuda shorts reaching her knees, and she would nod along with everything Eric said to us, give everything she had, never seeming to expect or demand more than what her body was capable of. Her disposition always seemed healthy and enviably normal. I was angry at my body instead of grateful, and negative about my performance instead of cheering my accomplishments.

When that was done, I blurted, "I'm so glad the jumping's over," at which point Eric said, "Time for vertical jumps."

The high jumps went pretty much the same as the long jumps, except I put on an even worse display. At the end of that test, Eric ordered, "To the squat machine!"

He said it just like that, as if we were off to save the world: *To the Batmobile!* We circled around the machine and I thought, *Yes—load bearing. I'm made for this.* Eric explained our job was to squat at the pace dictated by the metronome until we could no longer keep up, and then he set me up with 100 pounds on the bar. There was a red laser shooting out to tell me how low to go for the squat to count, and I lost myself until my legs wobbled and my knees creaked and Eric ran his finger over his throat: *You're finished.*

Some of the women struggled with 100 pounds on their shoulders. Some of us breezed through a few dozen squats.

All of us were exhausted. "Go home and rest," Eric said. "Day after tomorrow is the trailer pull. Trust me—you want to be fresh for that."

4

Shake me and my confidence

I pulled into the small, dusty lot at the edge of the Natick Woods. Everett, moving about as he always seemed to be, offered a distracted nod as I slammed my car door shut.

"*Hey.*"

I jumped at a voice behind me. "Hey! You scared me."

"Sorry," Elle giggled, reaching out and laying fingers lightly on my upper arm. "I'm a little nervous." Elle, it seemed, laughed when she was nervous. And happy. And tired. "Where is everybody?"

"Probably crushed under the weight of the trailer. Or lost in the woods," I replied. We headed over to the guys together, my nylon track pants whooshing as I walked. The weather was getting warm enough for shorts, but I still felt safer fully covered given all the sharp edges and wooden objects we came into contact with. There was no dress code here that we knew of, so the test subjects showed up in whatever clothes made us feel comfortable. "This is a completely normal thing to be doing on a Thursday afternoon. Right?"

Elle, in a white T-shirt and loose shorts, dark hair tied in a low, short pony, laughed some more as we watched Everett and Eric unloading a tarp-covered lump from the back of a pickup truck.

"There are only two trailers, so we'll be staggering the tests for the next few days until everyone goes," Everett called down to us.

I didn't see these so-called "trailers" we'd been told about, but harbored an image of being hitched to a double-wide and leaning into it like a captive ox as I hauled ass through the mud. The two guys pulled off the tarps to reveal two wooden wagon-like objects that weighted 110 pounds and could fit a toddler or two.

"Elle Montague. Come on up," Eric said.

"Where's the trailer?" I interjected.

No one responded. Eric picked up a strap attached to the wagon thingy and proceeded to wrap it around Elle's waist. That *couldn't* be it. I was underwhelmed. "It's smaller than I expected," I said with ill-advised cockiness.

"You'll go after Elle," Everett told me, pointing to the second wooden wagon.

Now belted in, Elle kicked the dirt with her boot to get a sense of her footing. And then she was off, with Eric following on a mountain bike. She disappeared into the trees.

"Stand facing the woods," Chris instructed me a few tense minutes later. I did, and I was now staring down an uneven wooded path that disappeared quickly after the first bend. Chris set the second trailer behind me, then reached around and clipped the belt on. The strap was padded in the front, and as Chris let go, I wiggled my hips to test its fit. Elle was galloping toward us now, her face paler than when she took off, tendrils of dark hair falling out of her ponytail.

"You ready?" Everett asked me.

I nodded. I wasn't, though. I couldn't settle into this odd experiment. I knew I could drag the trailer currently stuck to me, but I was fearful I couldn't drag it fast enough or hard enough or long enough. Elle was back, bent over, gasping, catching her breath.

"You made it look easy," I called over.

She stood upright. "It's not." For once, she wasn't laughing. "Keep control of it. It can tip if you're not careful."

Eric was back. He threw his leg over his mountain bike and said to me, "I'll be right behind you." Everett held the stopwatch this time. "Ready? Go!"

I took off. Or, more accurately, I *tried* to. Within a few strides it was clear this test wasn't only about strength or speed. With every step, the belt slammed me in the gut as the trailer jerked backwards. I hobbled along for a couple minutes out of synch, jogging and jerking, digging deep for patience and coordination. After a frustrating quarter mile I found my finesse, falling into a rhythm and taming the trailer so it went at my pace. I pushed harder; the wagon followed behind me like an obedient pup. And then, as soon as my confidence was reaching new heights, I came to a downward slope. I hit the crest and looked down. *Easy.* I started running, but the trailer's full weight began pushing me. I sped up to avoid being crushed or tripped up. The raggedy wooden nightmare bounced off rocks and tilted on its metal wheels, threatening to pull me down with it. I screamed and heard the crunch of Eric's bike behind me; he was there, but he offered no help.

Calm. Run. Steady. I forced myself to stay upright and in the moment. I slowed slightly, took shorter strides, and reached the bottom of the hill, at which point I sped up again. As I ran faster and faster, a thought fluttered in: *Is this what women in the military have to do? But with supplies in the trailer? And they're running for their lives?* Actually, the answer was yep—pretty much. USARIEM had developed this wagon to see if it could help soldiers transport heavier loads over mixed terrain, and we were here to try it out for them.

There was a flat stretch of open meadow up ahead. I made a beeline for it, and the trailer stayed with me. I wasn't even halfway done with this outrageous test. I made it to the edge of the wide-open space and soon realized "meadow" is another name for an un-mowed expanse choked with grass and wildflowers. I plowed in, and I instantly learned that dragging 110 pounds through two-foot weeds changes the game; the weight felt doubly heavy here. I felt nauseated and fought the urge to give up. In my peripheral vision I saw Eric pedaling his bike at a crawl next to me. I stopped, huffed, started again, sped up, and almost vomited with the pressure of the belt on my waist. Finally I made it across this field I would forever refer to as Hell

Meadow, back to the rocky, hilly dirt part of the course, and then did the same loop again, finally *galumping* toward the finish line with a rising anger. I wanted that trailer off of me. I jerked over the line with a flourish of Ev's stopwatch and the slow crunching of Eric's mountain bike tires. I hadn't shone. I was, at best, average.

I heard clapping and cheering as I crossed. I was miserable and panicked and didn't hide it. I glared and hyperventilated and ignored well-meaning people asking how I was, telling me I did well just to finish. *Oh, do shut up.* Why did I suck so terribly? I tore off my belt. I was in a fog of self-absorption. I heard distant calls of *Great job! It's hard, isn't it…are you OK? Sara?* I stalked off to the side of the lot to some bushes, doubled over, and began retching. I turned back to see everyone except Everett getting on with their business. He was watching with a thoughtful expression and his head tilted to the side. He didn't appear to be thrown by my display, nor was he judging me; he was simply observing and letting me be. Having calmed down a notch, I turned and walked slowly back toward them. "You're so upset," Everett said. "How interesting."

Two more cars pulled into the lot; the next round of victims had arrived. I caught Elle shooting a quick, blank look my way as if unimpressed and, perhaps, thinking of her children's tantrums. One of the team took note of this.

"You're worried about *this*?" he asked, tilting his head toward me. "This is nothing. Lacey Berner ran into a tree this morning."

I was coughing and swishing water in my mouth. I

swallowed too fast, and, through coughing, said, "She ran into a *tree*?"

"She ran into a tree," he said flatly. "She's fine."

I went back to work somehow, but didn't do much other than plan the next day's stories, then went home to find no message from Ford, and then I slept harder than I had in months.

What to eat? I scanned the menu at the Donut Depot drive-thru. It was backpack day and my stomach was in knots, but I knew things had to change with my diet. I had to eat to fuel my performance now—which meant choosing well *and* consciously timing my meals. I was bad at this on my best day, though I tended to follow the diet advice of the moment, which was low-fat everything. I cursed donuts in their deep-fried glory but allowed the occasional new-fangled fat-free cookies, those sweet cardboard ovals stuffed with hard paste and marketed as a healthy option. Frozen yogurt was health food, and cereal with skim milk or a bagel with a thin layer of jam were considered solid breakfast choices.

I couldn't think about food yet. I ordered coffee and headed to work. I cruised through the comfortingly bustling newsroom with an editor yelling *Where's my copy?* across the room as reporters worked the phones. I dropped my bag on my desk and handed a large coffee, no sugar, no dairy, to my friend Rebecca. "It's backpack day, right? Are you ready?" She asked, typing as she spoke, flitting her brown eyes up at me.

"No," I said. "I'm not remotely ready. I have a story due at noon, I have to be at the base before one-thirty, and at some point I have to eat *and* digest. And then I have to prance through the woods with the equivalent of both Olsen twins on my back."

Rebecca laughed, then did what she always did in her methodical, calm way. "You'll

be great. You're strong." She took a careful sip of her coffee. "What's the story?"

"Salmonella at McCladdens."

"Whoa. You'll never be able to eat there again. You know that, right? McCladden will drench your Caesar salad in arsenic dressing. I think his father brought the bricks for that place over from the old country himself."

I logged onto my computer, stared at the screen. "I am aware of this," I replied. I'd gotten a tip from a source and was about to follow it up with the health department. This story was not going to be good for me around town, even if it earned me points in the newsroom.

"How are the other women?" Rebecca asked. "The volunteers? What are they like?"

"They're nice," I replied. "I don't know how much we have in common. I'm not sure we'll be great friends, but we're getting along."

We both went back to chasing the news, and I managed to write and report a solid story on time. I tried to time my food right, grabbing a fast-food grilled chicken sandwich on a quick break, but I ate too late and felt heavy, like maybe I shouldn't have eaten at all given my nerves. I'd already begun to view the backpack test as the standard bearer, the ultimate test to show what women could actually *do* in the military as a practical task. The soldier I imagined myself standing in for would be transporting vital medical supplies, water, MREs (ready-to-eat meals in civilian-speak), bedding, and everything her unit would need to survive on the frontlines. She would be essential, and anxiety and digestion drama couldn't factor in.

I raced home to suit up. As I wriggled my socked feet into my boots while sitting on the edge of the double bed from 1-800-MATTRESS, I was reminded that Ford hadn't called since my unfriendly voicemail. This showed a lack of desperation. Maybe I wouldn't have to break up with him after all. Maybe when these scientists and trainers were done picking over the remains of my self-esteem, I would once again want someone to make out with.

Anyway, by one-thirty my stomach was bubbling and my heart was racing as I pulled into that dusty parking space at the edge of the wood. I stepped out of the car and Eric was already coming at me hoisting a 75-pound pack.

"You're late. You ready?"

"No."

"This is heavy," he grunted.

"Sorry. Yes." I looped my arms through the straps as he settled it on my back.

"Clip the belt around your waist." I did, and took a few shaky steps. *Dear God.*

"How does it feel?"

"Like you strapped your grandmother's grand piano to my back."

"Good. That's the idea."

He went to help the next woman. It was a quiet affair, the donning of the packs. There was shuffling of boots on gravel, loud exhaling, quick intakes of breath when a subject felt the full weight of the pack. A few *oofs.* The pack was an added weight I didn't need; it was a cement block sinking me into the ground. Everyone was ready quickly because the team didn't want us wasting one electron of energy off the course.

"Can we do this?" Amanda wondered aloud, trying and failing to stand up straighter.

"We can," Nadine said.

"Heck, yeah," Elle said.

"*Hell* yeah," I said, meaning it, at least right then.

The timer went, the *Ready, set, go!* was called and we were off, and soon after that was when I found myself passing Donna, the one carrying two-thirds of her own bodyweight, and wondering how the hell I was going to complete two miles. The only sounds were grunting, shuffling of boots over pebbles and packed earth. There was no speed fast enough. In military exercises you are usually given a time to hit, but we had no such limits. We were to go until our hearts exploded and our legs gave out. The test wasn't whether you could walk with the backpack on. It was how fast and how far you could go, and no matter who you are that's an end you'll never reach. To attempt to move faster each time is like trying to grasp infinity. Aiming for no time at all was like trying to wrap my fingers around a fog, pull it down, and lock it up. This test stirred up the biggest question of all, the one you can't help asking yourself as you're in the first quarter mile of hell: *Why? Why* am I doing this?

It wasn't for medals. Not for recognition or career advancement or a salary or glory. This one was for military women. As Everett had written in a report about the study, this woodland hike had direct combat implications, in that our 75-pound packs were standard weight for "approach marches." According to the unputdownable 2017 U.S. Army publication *Foot Marches*, "Commanders use tactical road marches and approach marches to rapidly relocate units within an AO [area of operations] to conduct combat operations….Approach marches are used when contact [with the enemy] is anticipated or intended." If women could be trained to lug heavy packs at an acceptable rate and distance, another flimsy argument to keep them out of combat would be dashed to smithereens. *That's* why we were pushing ourselves past the pain.

We had no fewer than six people watching out for us as we hiked, from Everett to Peter to Eric to Horace and Jo, our trusty grad-student interns. I almost fell a few times. If you don't lift your knees up high enough, if you're too fatigued to take a proper step, your boot's toe catches on an imperfection in the terrain and your burden will take you down. In the end, I came in close to the front of the pack. As I crossed the finish, I heard someone call out a time. I didn't take the number in because it would've meant little to me. I didn't know what was normal or what was excellent. I knew I wasn't first, and I was far from last, and that was OK—for now.

Afterward, I was overcome with an all-encompassing, full-body pain: My back hurt, I had a fresh batch of pink blisters forming, and my lungs ached. But I was alive and filled with such relief and pride that the agony begat something good: a high of endorphins and accomplishment colliding to form a sense of well-being I hadn't felt in a long time.

PART TWO

THIS IS HOW WE DO IT

5

This is how we do it

We'd survived the jumping to nowhere, the bruising box lifts, and the trailer pull through Hell Meadow. It was time for training, and I felt like I could breathe again. I imagined the future as a twelve-week break from humiliating weigh-ins, dreaded timers, knots in my stomach and men reminding me I had *one chance* to shine.

When I arrived for our first day, I was proved wrong on every count. First up: A weigh-in. "Sara," Eric commanded, pointing at the scale, which was out of its nook and standing like gallows in the center of the room.

Everything was different today. Just seven test subjects were in the great space, dwarfed under the exposed steel beams and harsh lighting, Chris was now training only the dawn A-Group, and Pete wasn't around. I hung back despite Eric's command. The others waited their turns tapping their feet or hugging themselves. It felt so public, like we'd been frog-marched to the town square to measure the pull of gravity on our bodies: *Hear ye, hear ye! Sally Smith weighs sixty and one-hundred pounds. Hear ye!* Eric was focused on his clipboard, completely unaware of the mental breakdown happening in front of him. I needed to get a grip, so I thought about people who had bigger problems, and I stepped up.

Eric moved the balance. I exhaled to unload the weight of air. He met my eyes coolly. "Same. Keep doing what you're doing. Next."

Fuck it. Fuck everyone and the tanks they rode in on. I was still in the two-hundreds, which, while only about thirty-four pounds on the surface of the moon, was an utterly ridiculous state of affairs considering I'd been running around for two weeks at Extreme Army Fat Camp. Eric was buried again in his clipboard and didn't seem to care. I was filthy with anxiety and shame and he was ticking off boxes. *Zero pounds.* It was a demon scratching at my brain with dirty, bent claws: *Zero pounds. Zero pounds.* ZERO. POUNDS. Who has two sore thumbs, works out hard, drinks (almost) no alcohol, eats no pizza, gets plenty of sleep for two full weeks and loses zero pounds? *This* chick. I mean, I'd eaten some grilled-chicken sandwiches, some Caesar salads from McCladdens to show Salmonella Seamus there were no hard feelings, and a few fat-free cookies over the week. I didn't count calories and I admittedly went out for a few drinks with the gang from the paper one night, but surely all this working out was supposed to cancel out a few minor indulgences?

The other women, I noted, didn't pay attention to my poundage. As the others stepped on one by one, the rest of us kept a polite distance. And finally, when Elle screamed something about losing a pound—"seven more to go! *Yeah*!"—the training to become the Army's most lethal female soldier began. Everett opened the thick file in his hand, pulled out a pack of stock paper, and gave one card to each of us.

"These are your weight records for the week. It lists each exercise you'll be doing," he told us. "You'll find alphabetized folders in the filing cabinet behind me." He turned and pointed. "Find your name and file your chart at the end of each day."

The weight cards contained a laundry list of exercises with exciting names like "back hyperextension" and "medium grip barbell press."

"You'll alternate routines," Everett continued. "On Mondays and Fridays, half of you will work on Regimen One, and the other half will do—"

"Let me guess," I interrupted. "Regimen Two."

"Exactly," Everett continued, not seeming to notice the dash of sarcasm in my voice. "Tuesdays and Thursdays, you'll swap."

"So what's Wednesday?" someone asked.

"Wednesday is Backpack Day," Everett said. "OK, let's move on."

"Backpack day?" I did not like the sound of Backpack Day.

Everett walked away. Eric was already there, waiting at

the bench press machine we'd thus far used only as a bench. Everett lay down on his back, and Eric spotted him from above as he demonstrated five quick reps. The weights were the size of car tires, but Everett lifted the bar like it was an oversized Q-tip. "You get the idea," Everett said. "On to upright rows."

We followed the leaders as they demonstrated each machine. There were the rows, the medium-grip barbell press, the back hyperextension, the squat machine, the dead lift and more. When we'd circled back to the cubicle area, Everett assured us, "We'll be around to guide you if you get stuck."

We all looked at each other. Were we supposed to just clamber onto a machine and start pumping?

"I'm never going to remember all this," someone sighed.

"I know what you mean," another said. She was staring at her page as if it might start barking directions at her. "This is…a *lot*."

We didn't have time to freak out further. "Let's go!" Eric pointed to Elle and me, and helped us come up with appropriate starting weights, while Everett walked the others to their first machines. The women's faces had blended together so far for the most part, but suddenly, as plates began clanging and grunts echoed in the room, I began to get to know them on sight, by voice, by presence.

Elle in particular became a more rounded character to me. In the early days I wasn't sure what to think about this loud, brash, bouncy individual. Sometimes, shy people are scared by bold ones. Sometimes, insecure people are threatened by confident ones. Elle was self-possessed and fearless. She had confidence like a tiger has prey drive. It was innate in her, and you didn't have to know her long to realize it. She was the first to spot me on the bench press and when she turned that energy on me, it was invigorating. I lay on my back and looked up. I curled my hands around the cold metal bar.

"I've got you," Elle said.

I kicked off the bench press with seventy pounds, which wasn't too hard—until my third set. I finished it, but I wouldn't be going up to seventy-five anytime soon. I looked around and saw the rest seemed to have found their grooves as well, though exercise fails did occur during our first hour of training: I forgot to clip the plates on Elle's bench press once and they clanked to the ground, missing my foot by an inch. One subject got stuck at the bottom of a squat she couldn't come out of. We learned quickly that the minute-and-a-half "rest" we were allowed between sets was no time at all. The guys stayed with us, corrected us, encouraged us, and showed us the ropes as many times as we needed to get it right. After I spotted Elle, too, she sat up and picked a number out of thin air.

"I'm going to bench my body weight before this is over," she said. "Think I can?"

"Why not?" I shrugged, though that sounded like a lot. "Let's go for it."

As I was calculating how many upright rows I had left for the day, Nadine shouted, "Done!" We all looked over.

"My arms feel like jelly, but I did it. And with ten minutes to spare."

Eric was not impressed. "Wrong," he shouted across the room. "You're running ten minutes *over.* The rest of you—get those final reps in."

I raced to the bench press and pushed out ten reps while Elle spotted me. It was one of the women yelling to another, "Don't you give up on me, solider!" that got me through the last painful reps, and I finished with laughter.

Five minutes later, we were all done, with an antsy Nadine waiting for us by the door. "What now?" She was doing slow side bends, her thin legs lost in baggy shorts. "Some stretching, maybe?"

Eric shook his head as he strode toward the door and beckoned for us to follow. "Now," he said, as he opened the front door, "we run."

Eric led us straight ahead past our little parking lot. I saw a pleasant, flat path winding off around the lake. I stopped and faced the water. Eric took a sharp left. *Oh hell, no.* He lined us up at the base of a steep hill rising up alongside our training room leading to the main part of the base where we hadn't yet ventured. I glared at that incline. This was my instant new enemy, possibly more so than the scale. *There is no way he is going to make us run up that thing after how hard we just worked.*

"You'll be doing a two-mile run—that's three loops around the base. Marion will lead the way for the first lap," Eric told us.

Everyone was quiet. I could hear the new leaves of

spring rustling and scratching all around us as the wind blew through. I tried to center myself as I did on my Walden Pond runs: No one here was judging me. It was two little miles—easy. I tried to think positive thoughts, but this hill, which was noticeably paved with a light, rough asphalt contrasting sharply with the slick black tar of the main parking lot, was too steep to make friends with.

"Why," I asked Eric, stalling like a pro, "would we *start* a run at the base of a hill with a 100 percent incline?" I kept my tone light, but I wasn't kidding. I whirled and pointed toward the path around the lake. "Why not go the other way?"

Eric was fiddling with his timer. "Because that way wouldn't hurt as much."

There it was, the smirk and a twinkle in the eye. He *got* my humor. He listened, he watched, and sometimes, he even laughed. He lost points, however, for forcing me to run.

I can't do this, I thought.

"Hey," Elle elbowed me. "You *can*."

I didn't mean to say it out loud. Eric raised his stopwatch and called out his now-familiar *Ready, set, go!* and off we went. Every step forward was an effort, an exercise in fighting gravity. Halfway up I was thinking about how I'd have to do this at least two more times today—and countless times for months to come. Elle and Marion pulled ahead immediately. I side-eyed Laurie, who seemed to be struggling but also determined as she kept her steps small and consistent.

At the top of the hill, which felt like half a mile but was probably less than 100 feet, I was dead last. I picked up my pace to catch up with the rest. Up ahead were drab, basic buildings, barracks and offices and common areas. We came upon a few soldiers chatting, some in civvies, most in uniform. As we jogged, more and more soldiers seemed to be milling about; it was starting to feel like a *lot* of soldiers, officers, and staff were on a late lunch break. I sped up.

I said out of the corner of my mouth as I joined the main pack, "Is it just me, or are we being watched?"

Someone grunted back, "It's not just you."

I waited a few beats. "They're not cheering us on," I huffed. I wanted to stop *so bad*; my heels hurt and my quads were almost out of juice. My bra was not offering sufficient support. Note to self: Get down to Filene's lingerie department *stat*. "They think we're a joke."

I shot a look to Marion. Her steely eyes were trained on the path ahead of her. She remained at the front, upped her pace, maybe heard us chit-chatting, maybe not. I saw a guy smirking. It felt like high school, but I told myself I was being paranoid; we were working our asses off to help the military. Surely these people wouldn't mock us for such valiant efforts? *Of course they would*, a logical voice in my head argued. I'm sure many believed we didn't belong here. We were poseurs dropping into their lives for a visit, and when it was over we'd leave, safe and sound, while they continued serving our country. I could see the last building up ahead, then a bend in the road that led back down along the riverbank. As we passed the last of our "fan" club, we were alone again, and my thoughts turned back to the task at hand.

Pain. Pain. Pain. Pain. Shit. Pain. No more. I can't. I stopped and walked.

Laurie and Amanda passed me. I was officially last. I choked up. I was about to cry like a spoiled, weak brat. *I never signed up to run. I wasn't told I'd have to weigh myself publicly. I can't handle this.*

Laurie was ahead of me, her tiny, slow steps never ceasing. "Come. On," She huffed and puffed. "You. Can. Doooh. It."

Elle heard this, and began jogging in place, letting Nadine and Marion take the lead alone. "Come on, Sara! Let's go!" Elle shouted back to me while she waited for me to catch up. "Two more laps and we're done!"

I wanted to yell at her to get away from me. What *was* it about running that turned me into Beezlebub? They all kept going. All of them except Donna. So far she had been The Quiet One, and all I knew about her is that she worked hard and had freckles on her nose, round glasses and a short haircut somewhere between a bob and a pixie. Now, out of nowhere, she fell in beside me. Her dastardly ploy worked. I'd be damned if I was going to hold anyone else back, so I picked up my feet and kept up with her. I knew why she was there. I knew how I must look: like a petulant child. I started running faster.

Soon we were back at the bottom of that hill. I noted again how light its pavement was against the blacktop of our little parking lot, as if someone had tacked it on as an afterthought, and it reminded me of cement or concrete. That day a nemesis was born: Cement Hill. *Die, Cement Hill*, I thought as I approached it. I was about to walk again when I caught Eric staring at me like he could read my mind. I revved up, and a few others followed suit. But not Laurie, who was now coming up behind me. She kept up her tortoise routine: slow, steady, never giving up, never seeming to indulge in negativity.

"Let's make it to that building," Donna said as we hit the main drag again, pointing at a bunch of buildings that all looked the same. "Make it there and then you can stop."

We made it to the building, which turned out to be the farthest one. "Just make it to that tree. You see that tree? Then we can stop." I made it to the tree. Donna turned and smiled at me.

On that day when my sneakers first slapped the pavement on Cement Hill, with Donna spurring me on, I let the *I can'ts* fade. When I rounded the last bend, I saw Elle yelling and raising her arms at the finish line. I broke into a full run and crossed the line at the base of that same hill, and I cursed its name. "Fuck you, Cement Hill."

"Cement Hill?" Eric repeated, eyes narrowed, then closed for a quick flash. "OK. Cement Hill it is. See you tomorrow."

Yes. *Maybe.* I stalked back to the training room, unable to figure out why I was my own worst enemy. Maybe the peaceful solitude of Walden Woods hadn't been so good for me after all. Maybe I'd gotten too comfortable with no accountability beyond the trees. They never judged me. But they never pushed me, either. They let me sink into their branches with a long exhale, then let me go, but in the end they got me nowhere special.

Elle was spotting me again on the bench press the next day, and as I fought with a 75-pound bar, she blurted, "Something isn't right."

"Uh, you're right! Hello? Uh…help…*Elle…*" I was in danger of being crushed under the weight of the barbell.

"Oh, durn it! Sorry!" she laughed as she put four fingers on the barbell to save me from strangling myself with a metal bar. "I'm here. You've got this. Come on! Lift it!"

But no, I *didn't* have it. I'd upped the weight I was lifting too far, too fast. My left hand was collapsing, so Elle brought it back up to the holders with a *clink-clunk*. "Does anyone else think something is off in this room?" Elle inquired to no one in particular.

"Nothing is *off*," Eric answered her from across the room. "Everything is as it should be—except there's no one lifting weights. Let's *go*."

Elle moved on to another set of rows. Someone started humming one of the biggest songs of the year, "This Is How We Do it." Elle hummed along as she hit the back machine again, followed by more abs work. And on her last move, she sat up with an "A ha!" And then nothing. She hopped off, toweled her neck down, then ambled over to Eric, who was surveying from the margins, his hawk eye on his subjects' form. I decided Elle must have figured out what was allegedly "off" around here and solved it somehow.

"Done!" she sang. "I'm ready for a run. Or whatever surprise you have in store for us."

Eric swept his eyes around the room. I saw the same scene he surely did: a bunch of exhausted, sweaty, sore, bruised women. Amanda was shaking her arm out like she was trying to slough off the soreness. Nadine was sitting on the bench, head between her legs. Elle stretched one of her quads.

"You're finished," Eric said. "Go home, get some rest, and come back tomorrow ready to work."

I walked into the training room Wednesday already sore from a two-day week to find the guys bustling about, studying their ubiquitous clipboards or fiddling with backpack straps, then turned when Elle burst in—you always knew when Elle entered a room—and announced, "I figured out the problem. We need music. I mean we need music *every day*," she demanded.

"Today is backpack day. We'll be outside," Eric said as he weighed a backpack. "The only music you'll be hearing is the sound of my voice telling you to go faster. I can put a tune to it if you want."

And then Elle uttered what would become her catchphrase for as long as I knew her, always uttered through a wince of disappointment and a laugh: "Oh, *maaaaaan*!" The rest of the women trickled in. Marion was the last to arrive that day, and I watched through the door as she bid goodbye to a tall man with the close cut of a young Army private. I saw him wave and walk away, his stride long and his posture like a board.

"Let's go!" Eric called to us.

He led us past the backpacks and out the door.

"This is light," Marion proclaimed as she tightened the belt around her waist at the start line by the lake. "Two miles will be nothing."

She was the only one with a pack on. "Wait," I said to Eric, his stopwatch poised. "Isn't it kinda hard to have Backpack Day without the backpacks?"

"You're going without one today," Eric said, fiddling with his stopwatch.

"But Marion has one."

"Because she's a soldier and she's used to it. We know what we're doing," Eric said. "Trust us."

Trusting a man blindly was not my forte. It was not in my blood. But in this case, I was being asked to walk miles without any added weight, so I acquiesced. Everett finished clipping on his own pack and informed us, "You'll carry next week, anywhere from twenty to thirty-five pounds. You'll be going five miles, and your goal is to complete the course in under seventy-five minutes. Those who succeed today will have weight added next week, anyone falling below that will remain the same, and those who struggle to finish—or don't finish—will have their weight reduced."

"Do *what*?" Elle laughed.

"Fuck that," I answered.

"So are you saying we should run?" Nadine asked.

"Not necessarily," Everett shook his head. "You need to get the feel of five miles in your legs. Hike, walk fast, keep up your pace to hit the seventy-five minutes, but don't try too much too soon."

Eric clicked his stopwatch and told us to go, and we walked together as Ev guarded the fringes like a papa bear. It was getting hot now. Memorial Day was coming soon, to be followed by summer, at which point I would have to wriggle myself into some sort of bathing apparatus, so it was just as well I was doing a five-miler today. With testing over, I was able to appreciate the mild weather, the light glinting off the lake's surface, the quiet on our side of the base.

We weren't here to make friends, and so far we'd been focusing on the work above all else. That five miles was when I truly started to get to know the C-Group women. Donna, my running friend, didn't have to work hard to keep me honest that day. I was happy to enjoy a long, fast walk with no expectation of a sprint. Nadine stared down the miles in front of her like she wanted to break into a run *so bad*. Amanda, wild curly black hair blowing free, had a curious, kind, even disposition. Laurie, with little athletic experience, was unapologetically out of her element but had a natural fortitude and was taking to it well.

And, of course, there was Elle. As we marched I asked her flat out how she stayed so buoyant through all of this. She seemed to know what I was really asking. "You know what?" she said. "My mama always said, 'Elle, you're no better than anyone else—and no worse. Don't you ever forget that.' And you know what?"

"You never forgot that," I guessed.

"Never," she smiled.

"You're from the South?"

"Well, now, depends who you ask. Macon's from Texas. I grew up in Florida."

To avoid thinking about the hiking boots rubbing against my raw skin, I asked, "So you're married, huh? What's that like?"

I wanted to say, *Why did you do that to yourself?* Where other young women saw bows tying up their happy ever after, I saw chains. Where was the fun in staying in every night with the same guy? Where was the excitement in his morning breath and moods? You go to bed—he's there. You wake up—he's there. Furthermore, how could you do anything interesting with your life while two little humans were pulling at your pantlegs? Why give up your freedom?

"Aw, *maaaan*," Elle trilled. "He's my best friend. Macon's been my man since we were eighteen."

"That's sweet," Laurie said.

I still didn't get it—how could a man be a best friend *and* someone who leaves you breathless? With me it had always been either/or: I went faint with lust and adoration, or I saw him as a comfy pal, like a favorite old shoe. Ford somehow seemed to be lingering in the space between. Everyone was quiet as we focused on walking faster. As if she'd read my mind, Elle asked me, "What about you? Is there a guy?"

Fuck it. I decided to tap into the wisdom around me. "Yes and no," I said.

"Let's pick it up," Eric commanded.

"Ooh. Wait for me," Amanda said, striding up alongside me.

I told them about Ford, and how he was floating along in a vague career of "sales and marketing" and I wasn't sure he was creatively ambitious enough for me. About how he was nice but not too nice; how he was dependable but never crowded me; and how I felt crowded by even *one* phone call that came too close to the last. I explained I liked being with him and even sometimes got one little fluttering butterfly, *but:* "I think there's something wrong with me," I said, fully believing it. This was not normal. A normal young single lady doesn't overthink a guy like Ford. (Does she?). "What do I do? Am I being neurotic? Do I keep hanging out and let it take care of itself, or snuff it out now?"

I was ready to snuff it like a warm fire before bedtime because with no one caring enough to tend to it, it could burn your house down. Nadine fell in and listened intently as I huffed and puffed through the story.

"I get it," Elle said. "I don't know if you should snuff anything yet. It's a balance. But I think you'll know, Sara. When it happens, you'll *know.*"

That's what they all say. "I hope so," I replied to be polite.

"If you haven't had actual butterflies more than once—what did you say, you had them one time?" Elle pressed.

"I didn't count each individual butterfly," I said as I sped up, at which point I realized certain things made me able to run. Ask me about my weight or my dating life and suddenly I'm a keen marathoner. "I don't know. I had three butterflies? Two times, maybe?"

"Just two times?" Nadine confirmed as she passed. "Let go. Just uncurl your fingers and fall. Hanging on will only prolong the agony. Trust me."

Trust me. Nadine had been married and knew her stuff, I figured. OK, I thought. I will. I decided to trust these people I'd volunteered to hang out with for seven months. I also wondered what made Nadine say that, because it seemed to me she was speaking from experience. Donna stayed silent through our discourse, seeming more interested in the cracks in the pavement than in this particular conversation.

"What do you do, Nadine?" I'd heard she was a sharp businesswoman, but so far she hadn't talked much about her profession.

"I sell insurance," she said. "Are you covered? I mean, do you have *enough* insurance?"

"I don't know," I replied. *Was* I underinsured? Was I *totally* protected from everything I could be protected from?

"We'll talk," Nadine assured me. "I bet you I can get you cheaper car *and* renter's insurance."

"Renter's insurance?"

Nadine tried to hide her horror, but she only half-succeeded.

Everett appeared out of nowhere. "Let's go a little faster," the scientist with the floppy hat said. "We're going too slow to make seventy-five minutes."

We obeyed. When we made it to the finish, Marion and her mystery man met up again, alternately grinning like fools in a nineties rom-com then talking seriously, intimately about something as they walked away, back to their regular Army lives.

We showed up on Thursday closer than we'd been on Tuesday. Friendships form fast with mutual suffering, and they grow deeper with shared secrets. I could feel the difference. There was a warmth in the room and a new familiarity that suddenly made the work easier. There was also beautiful music: Boston's 94.5 FM was playing on a boombox that had appeared out of nowhere. Elle played with the volume. "Who did this?"

"Everett," Eric replied.

Later, I looked over at Elle on the sit-up machine, humming and smiling as she absorbed herself in song.

At the end of our bench presses and pulls and sit-ups and squats that day, Eric corralled us. "Time for sandbag runs," he said. "While you were all lifting and squatting, our interns were outside preparing a treat for you. Follow me."

We walked outside and saw a course strewn with misshapen brown lumps. Our two unsympathetic interns, Jo and Horace, were standing proudly over a row of stuffed burlap bags. "There are five piles," Eric boomed. "You'll take turns running them back and forth from the line."

"How many times do we run it?" Laurie, ever earnest and eager, asked.

"You run until I tell you to stop," Eric replied. "I want to see you give *everything*."

I took a closer look at the bags. "Do *what*?"

"FUCK THAT!" came a chorus in response.

"You know," a not-amused Eric said, tilting his head and regarding us all with that cool gaze, "my other groups don't complain like you. They actually respect me."

"They sound really boring," I retorted.

Eric turned his narrowed eyes on me. Then he raised his famous stopwatch and yelled *Ready, set, go!* Scooping up fifty pounds of untamed sand is harder than it sounds. Sand is slithery, ornery dead weight, as it's meant to be. I tried to hug the bag to myself, but it slipped through my arms. I tried to carry it like a baby, but I couldn't hold it. I watched Nadine throw it against her shoulder, then copied her.

Elle and Marion were engaged in some sort of unspoken competition. They were going to kill themselves before they let one outdo the other. We were giving *everything.* By the time Eric yelled *stop*, we were panting, spent, done in. We were all grinning, too—every last one of us. Everyone raised up a hand and as we walked it off, we gave each other high fives. Sandbags were another thing we'd never done before; you don't encounter those at the local gym.

Like everything the team put before us, the sand was in our arms for a purpose, and we carried it into the future. The cold barbells we wrapped our warm fingers around, the weights we dropped on our toes, the blisters stinging as we strained our shoulders running with dead weight, it was all meant to assist future military women—in and out of combat roles.

When sandbag runs were over that day, I sauntered by Eric, wiping myself down. "Was that *everything* enough for you?"

He shrugged. Something was off with him, I thought. He seemed tired. Grumpier, distracted. Not interested in taking any of my crap, even it if my crap *was* clever and adorable.

Catherine: 2014

Catherine Afton was nervous and excited when she landed at her chosen university—until she attended her first ROTC orientation. It was, she says, the shock of her life. This wasn't high school anymore. She wasn't the captain of any sports teams, nor was she number one in any class (yet). The rules of her entire life had changed, and she was wrong-footed from the moment she arrived.

"Indoc," or new-student indoctrination, teaches the importance of teamwork and unit cohesiveness and introduces cadets to life in the military, to discipline, to the new way they do their hair and wear their sleeves. They practice things like "warrior toughness" and physical fitness, and with indoc came challenges Catherine wasn't used to.

"They were telling me I wasn't good enough," she recalls, "and I was really buying into it."

On top of all of that, things were falling apart back home; her parents had recently separated and Catherine could expect to return for the winter holidays to a new version of the family she'd left in August. The girl who had succeeded at nearly everything she'd tried, whose family was always rooting for her and giving her space to thrive, grew so overwhelmed that one day, as she walked through campus, she felt sobs building in her. She spotted a thick, lush bush up ahead. Its leaves could shield her, and its safe harbor seemed to be her only option if she didn't want passersby seeing the unraveling of Catherine Afton. She dove in and cried alone, sobbing quietly as twigs brushed her face and scratched her neck.

"I crawled into a bush and cried my eyes out. 'Maybe I *can't* do this. Maybe they're right.' I felt very confused, and I remember I was just falling apart underneath this bush in the first week of school and the first week of ROTC," she says now.

She soon pulled herself together and headed back to her dorm room—to research ways out of the bargain she'd made. "I thought, OK, I could go to my safety school if I drop out of ROTC…and then I can take out some loans. I walked to a nearby coffee shop and wrote a bit of stuff down. In the end I thought, I'm not taking on two-hundred-fifty K in debt. Not a chance."

This latest list woke her up like an ice bucket dumped over her head. She made the decision over weak coffee and strong resolve that she would take whatever the ROTC officers dished out. A little voice inside her asked, *Can I really get through this?* Another answered, *Only if you don't give up.*

Fast forward a couple months, and Catherine Afton was pedaling hard, then coasting over the bumpy cobblestones of the college town's deserted streets, wind in her hair and a peace about her. She owned that usually busy stretch for a short time as the first light of dawn seeped over the horizon. It was her favorite time of day during those first months when she finally sank into the culture of ROTC. She loved waking up so early when the streets were empty; she could bike in the middle of the road because no one was there. Rising before the sun was always worth it.

She'd become accustomed to the rhythms of life as a young military candidate. After the self-given pep talk that day in the coffee shop, Catherine had allowed herself more time to adjust. It would be hard, but she had done hard things before, so why should this be any different? Before long, she began to form tight bonds within the program, and everything got better.

"I found a family in ROTC," she recalls. "I needed warmth and connection and that was huge. Upperclassmen were so supportive. I made a bunch of mistakes, and they helped smooth it over."

She stuck with it, because even so young she knew that if you don't plow through the challenges, you'll never see what's on the other side. She felt the fear and she did it anyway. That is what courage is, after all; acknowledging the terror spreading inside you and refusing to let it feed off of you. She starved the fear until it died. Still, she couldn't have known then how much tougher it was going to get.

6

One of us

Eric Lammi was not thriving. The single sportsman should've been a carefree man-about-town, but he was growing tired of driving eighty miles round-trip to a full-time job with high stakes. The commute from Lunenberg, a town settled in the year 1718, population 9,000, a place that would serve as a perfect Colonial American movie set, was starting to get to our trainer.

He was living in his family's lake house and building a new septic system with his father on weekends. And then, every Monday, it was back to the long journey to work to hear people like me whine about Cement Hill. A few weeks into the study, Eric approached Everett in his office on the base. "Something has to change," he said.

Everett stopped what he was doing. "Oh?"

"I can't do this right if I'm driving so much. You know anyone who would do a temporary lease?"

Everett gave his trainer his full attention. "Funny you should ask," he replied.

Eric was a nomad at heart, even if he didn't go out of his way to describe himself as one. Possessions, big houses, commitments, roots, office jobs, these were anathema to him. They did not factor into his value system at the time. Granite countertops and children and the best schools were not dreams he harbored at age forty. He wanted to explore the world and meet people and do important things like coach athletes to greatness. A life spent around athletics was his most precious currency, his personal wealth, and his oxygen.

You didn't have to be a member of a championship team to get Eric's whole heart when he trained you, either. That was the beauty of sport; Eric could coach the Hopkinton High School girls track team and watch them win seven outdoor State Divisional Titles and five straight All-State Titles, and that received as much of his relentless dedication as the U.S. Army or the Olympic trials. He expected the same effort from everyone—girls, men, women, boys.

This Army thing was another stop on the long, winding journey Eric was on, and he intended to immerse himself like there was literally no tomorrow—because for him tomorrow was a haze. The decathlete we literally looked up to five days a week began life as an unlikely track star. Those who excel at this test of athleticism are widely considered the best of the best, as King Gustav V of Sweden famously told Jim Thorpe after he won the decathlon in 1912: "You, sir, are the world's greatest athlete." One obvious reason for that is competitors must master *ten* events such as the discus, javelin, long jump and pole vault.

Growing up in the North Shore area of Massachusetts in the small town of Topsfield on the Ipswich River, Eric, who is of 100 percent Finnish extraction, took to sports almost as soon as he could walk, but the size of his body was slow to catch up with the breadth of his enthusiasm.

"I was tiny," Eric told me. "I was five-three, eighty-six pounds in eleventh grade."

His small stature didn't prevent him from performing on the field, the track or the court. It simply gave his school's coaches an excuse not to give him a chance. "I was a really good basketball player," Eric says. "I played in the town league and was a starting guard, but when I got to high school they put on a one-hour tryout and cut all the short kids. I'll never forget it. I feel that I would have been one of the top two basketball players in the school."

Eric had a shot at track, though, and he seized it. His father was a long-jumper and Eric found he could soar higher and farther than nearly anyone in town: At four-foot-eight as a freshman, he could jump over his head. It was, he said, one long growth spurt that got him near the place where I met him. "I grew six inches all at once. By the end of junior year I was probably five-nine, and when I graduated high school I was six-one."

Young Eric found success in the state high jump and triple jump in the seventies, then snagged a place at the

University of Maine. "I high jumped there, longjumped and triple jumped, and was one of the top in New England. I was captain of the team and set school records and conference records," he explained. "I wasn't at a national level, but I always wanted to do the decathlon."

He wanted to do it at the expense of any sort of settled life, knowing he'd never fit into the box he was supposed to. When he graduated from UMaine—pre-med with a degree in zoology—the last thing he wanted was to put a suit and tie on and get a nine-to-five job, and so, "I jumped in a decathlon, did very well, then floundered around, did a few more, and did OK."

But he was still young and unfocused, and time, as it does, moved faster than he did and he saw his dream start to slip away. "I wasn't really training right. I was mixing it with traveling and partying. It was 1982 when I decided *OK.* This is my last chance. I was getting into my mid-to-late twenties. I really wanted to do it. I could run a five-minute mile without any training. I could beat everybody in sprinting except a real sprinter."

And so Eric, a walking dichotomy of commitment-phobia and unrelenting dedication, reached out and pulled the dream out of the sky like a kite before the wind could carry it out of reach. "I went to Colorado and trained for the decathlon," he said simply, reducing an incredible feat to one sentence. "And I made it to the Olympic trials as one of the top people in the country."

He gave the same *everything* he was always asking of his test subjects. It wasn't enough. Eric has had asthma most of his life and suffered chronic sinus infections.

"Unfortunately, I was sick at the trials and didn't end up finishing it," he says. "I wasn't expecting to make the team. Just to make it to the trials is a goal for a lot of people. You know you won't make it, you're *just* a level below. Fewer make the Olympic team in track than play pro football."

When he wandered into Ev's experiment, Eric still hadn't found a niche for himself. Even if he thought he didn't need somewhere to settle down, fate was coming for him. Everett came through for Eric after that talk about his commute and offered him a spot in his rental property. Mary Desmond of A-Group and her roommate Lisa were home when Eric pulled up to their two-family house in his silver Nissan Sentra. He would be taking the third room in their half of Everett's home; another roommate had just left and the women were looking for a new one.

Mary, who trained with Chris Palmer in A-Group and was far less enamored of Eric than I was, answered the phone when he called to confirm there was a place for him and told her, "OK. I *guess* I'll move in." Mary shrugged and told him he was welcome, but thought to herself, *Sure, buddy. Don't do us any favors.*

Eric unloaded his car, entered his new home for the first time, and followed Mary to his room. She meant to offer to help carry in the rest of his things, but there was nothing to take. Everything he needed he had on him. He moved in with a small gym bag, a sleeping bag and his javelin. When he was safely ensconced in his room, Mary turned to Lisa. "What is that stick he brought in here? Did this guy just move into our apartment with camping gear and some kind of spear-fishing apparatus? This should be interesting."

Eric slept on the floor on a camping pad, figuring he'd be fine for the duration of the study, and then he'd move on like he always did. But before long, one of his B-Group volunteers, Beatrice, learned of his situation and wouldn't have it. She got on the case and together with a few other volunteers found Eric a mattress, making sure he had somewhere comfortable to sleep while he trained the women who wanted to make history.

In the midst of dealing with bruises and blisters and tears and doubts and fears, I was beginning to craft my first article about the study. I wrestled with how to do justice to the personal experiences of forty-six women in 1,800 words, which is impossible, but I was too inexperienced to know it.

I spoke to my C-Group friends first. I noted Laurie often asked thoughtful questions and seemed to attack Cement Hill with a positive attitude, a quality I admired. Laurie Masten Scott appeared to have her life in perfect order: two daughters, a loyal husband with a stellar career in journalism, a house in the suburbs, and an easy peace about her. When I sat down with her and asked what made her submit to this insane trial, her answer surprised me. "It had been one of the hardest years of my life," she replied. "I had to do *something*, or I was going to lose it."

At thirty-six, Laurie was the oldest test subject in the

study and never should have been on Cement Hill with us at all. The scientists had set clear parameters from the outset: Volunteers over thirty-two years of age need not apply. But Laurie refused to be underestimated based on a number. She'd written letters, made phone calls and demanded to be excepted and accepted.

At the time she'd read about the experiment she was lost, and had gripped onto this odd endeavor to anchor herself to the next phase of her life. Her husband's job as a reporter for the *Christian Science Monitor* had taken them to exotic places, and repatriating had been a rocky process. "We had just returned to the U.S. after being in Mexico City for four years, and before that Australia, and before that New York City," Laurie, who had been teaching English while in Mexico, told me. "We were settling in Framingham, and my life hadn't started yet as far as work, so Dave came home one day with this article about the strength study and said, 'Look at this, Laurie!'"

I laughed a little, because if a man showed me an article about how I could exercise for seven months he'd be risking his own health.

"Showing me the study wasn't about working out," she laughed too. "It was about what he and I refer to as our Year from Hell. He was just coming off being a foreign correspondent being wined and dined, and I was coming off seeing the world, and we were both having an identity crisis. He knew I needed something to get excited about and dig deep on. I'm always into 'you go, girl' stuff," she added. "Dave knows that I love him and all the men in my life, but I raise my children to know a woman needs a man like a fish needs a bicycle. I'm raising them with the idea you have to be your own strong individual woman even if you're in love and married. Dave knew this would speak to my heart. He was absolutely right."

She read the article, and then "I called Everett and Pete immediately. I thought, this is *awesome*. I met the scientists and they said they liked my attitude, so they upped the maximum age for me."

In the end, my first article didn't go deep on any of the test subjects. I set the scene and described the pain, jubilation, victories and struggles of our most dramatic tests. Andrea and another editor had first crack at it, and the night editing team—hard at work putting out the morning edition—polished it and packaged it up. For one editor in particular, Rus Lodi, this project was interesting in more ways than one—his two sisters were Army officers.

The story ran on the front page of the *Middlesex News* on Thursday, May 25 with a photo of C-Group enduring our first five-mile hike with the headline *Tough as Males* splashed across it. I drove to the base the day it ran, and I could see a copy of the newspaper in O'Hara's booth. He betrayed nothing as I drove up. No congratulations—but no frown this time, either.

When I walked into the training room, my friends greeted me with smiles and praise. Everett held a copy in his hand and it crinkled loudly as he gave me a hug. "I loved the story," he smiled.

I was proud of the piece, but loathed the image of me striding at the front of the pack.

I said, *I look lumpy.*

C-Group said, *No you don't. You look cute.*

They didn't say, *Don't worry! We'll smooth down your lumps with all this training. We'll make you thin.*

They said, *Stop it. You look great.*

That was the moment I felt safe with them, unconditionally.

7

Power, pleasure, pain

I was a civilian with at least one extremely annoying thing in common with soldiers: Blisters. Those innocent-looking, liquid-filled blobs can take you down and out before you know it. As an article on the Army's own website points out, what some might call "just a blister" can debilitate you, develop into a dangerous infection, and, "as one of the most common injuries among active duty military, friction blisters can have a notable adverse impact to military readiness."

On the next backpack day, Everett loaded me up with twenty-five pounds. It felt fine at first but after the first two miles, I began swearing liberally and loudly. This was no tantrum, mind you; anyone could see I was in total agony.

"I'm in total agony!" I shouted.

Pete Frykman was right behind me. They were always watching over us on bikes, on foot, with backpacks and water bottles. "If it's that bad, you should stop."

"But that will mess up my time." *Huff, puff, huff, puff.*

With every step I took, it felt like my boots were rubbing another layer of skin off. I was biting my lip for a few yards, keeping quiet, wondering if I could tolerate it. Everyone else was moving—and not complaining.

"It's fine," I grunted after a few beats.

Near the end, I wanted to cry, and then I wanted to throw up from the pain. Pete was with me again as I swore once more.

"You're not OK," he observed. "Stop if you need to."

Not a chance. I kept (relatively) quiet after that. Pete faded out to trail someone else, and I eventually fell in step with Donna and Marion. I said to Marion, "All this stuff we've been doing—it must be what basic training is like, right?"

Marion pressed on. "This is nothing like basic training."

Oof. "Oh…ah…right. Sorry—I didn't mean any disrespect," I huffed and puffed, trying to keep up with her and ashamed of minimizing female soldiers' pain. "Of course this is nothing compared to what you go through. I'm an idiot."

"This," Marion said as she pulled ahead of me and left me in the dust, "is much harder."

By the last lap, everything hurt and I was desperate to pee. I was in tears from the blisters, but they were silent rivulets streaming down my red face; there would be no tantrums. Not on backpack day.

They tried to help me with the blisters over the

following weeks. The team came up with moleskin, band aids, gauze pads, and new hiking boots. I tried special, thick military grade socks. None of it helped. My C-Group friends would circle around as I peeled off a sock to find new blisters—sometimes filled with blood—under my sock. "How can you even walk?" Donna asked on one particularly gruesome backpack day when strips of bloody skin were hanging off my ankles. "When your feet are shredded like that?" She shook her head with a mixture of horror and wonder.

I didn't know how; I just did it. I tore a hanging piece off, wrapped my foot back up, and got ready to put on my pack and head out to the course. I was officially emotionally attached to the study. I loved the routine, the hiking course with its view of the lake, the women, my trainer, the way the two scientists would push us hard and the careful way they'd watch over their precious human test subjects protectively and unconditionally. If we were hurt, they were hurt. If we failed, they failed.

On my way out that day, hobbling to my favorite red backpack, Nadine said to me, "Even with all that blood and pain you're getting back out there. Wow."

I choked up hearing Donna and Nadine say those things; I spent much of the study writing about others' bravery, and my own failings. I thought about how so often women, especially of my generation and before, seem to make a lifetime of self-deprecation and an almost manic modesty, of putting ourselves down, and I started to think maybe we should stop. Maybe I should stop. The world is hard on us all, and judges us harshly. We can only hope to meet the souls who lift us up in the midst of it so we can make it through in one piece.

The official start of summer was a hair's breadth away. Schools were letting out, college graduations were over, and we'd gotten down to hard-core training. On one particularly warm day, a woman I *thought* I recognized wandered into our training room at one-thirty. I gave her the side-eye from afar, and watched as Eric greeted her. C-Group drew our weightlifting cards from the cabinet and moseyed over.

"Everybody," Eric called out. "This is Jean. She's a refugee from D-Group, and she needs a new home. Let's welcome her to C-Group."

"Welcome!" Laurie waved, and smiled warmly at the new girl. "It's nice to have you with us."

"Hi, Jean," we all echoed, then peppered her with questions.

"You'll love C-Group."

"What made you leave D?"

"What's your—"

Eric stopped us short. "Save it for later. We have work to do."

I never like change, especially when I have no warning and no control over it. I sized up this Jean person who would add an unknown variable to our delicate C-Group balance, and saw a calm woman with a shy smile, a scrunchy holding back her feathered brown hair, and a relaxed lope as she moved from machine to machine.

Eric decided that day would be "core" day, which I was learning involved anything that wasn't an arm or a leg. The abs machine was easy enough—hook your ankles under a padded thing and do a shit-ton of crunches—but I was struggling with the weird back contraption.

"I *suck* at the vertical," I lamented as I stared at my card and then at the machine in front of me. "I don't think I'm doing it right."

Eric came over with the cynical look I was growing used to. "The *vertical?*" He frowned. "That is not the 'vertical.' I'll show you what a vertical workout would look like."

He stood in place, arms glued to his sides like a Fisher Price figure, leaned backward stiffly one millimeter, then forward two, then backward in a few tiny jerks.

I laughed until I cried. He said, "Get on the *horizontal* machine and I'll show you. It's not hard."

I got on the soft cushioned bench and laid on my stomach. "Tuck your feet under the pads behind you. Hands on your neck, elbows out. Good. Now, without arching your back, move up and down, using your hips like hinges. Kind of like an upside-down sit-up."

He stood close, placing one hand on my lower back and another on my shoulder. His hands were huge, warm, comforting.

"Lean back. That's it." He held gently on to me for the first rep, then let go so I could finish on my own. A thought popped into my head: *Don't let go.* "You've got it. Good. Now you're the first person in history to get a vertical workout."

"You do realize you're not as funny as you think," I hit back.

"You're right. I'm funnier," he deadpanned, then walked away to help someone else.

At the end of weight training, Eric directed us back to the start line on Cement Hill. I'd vowed to keep the drama to a minimum, but I felt sick as he raised his stopwatch of doom. My blisters were still bad, and the heat never helped.

"It's OK," Donna whispered next to me.

Eric shouted *Go!* and the others were halfway up before I even hit my stride. I ran the first lap, but the pain—mental and physical—kicked in. I stopped to tie my shoe to give myself a quick break. I moved each tie slowly and created perfect, careful loops on both shoes. Out of the corner of my eye I saw two men in uniform staring at me. I finished, stood up, and gave them a weary half-smile as they passed.

They both sneered. "You signed up for this," one of the soldiers hissed. "Guess you better deal with it." They shook their heads and kept walking.

I saw Jean, in the middle of the pack running alone, take note of what had happened. I ran as fast as I could away from them, joining the middle of my pack all the way back to the base of Cement Hill. Jean was there, and gave me a nod. Her face said, *Fuck those guys.* I smiled back, and finally remembered where I knew her from: We'd suffered together on the VO2 max test. I *knew* I liked her.

When we finished the run, Elle waited for us all to catch our breath, then followed us as we headed to the training room to grab our things. "The weekend's coming up," she said. "Macon's away on business. I have the big old house to myself—I think it's time we had a little fun. Whaddaya say?"

We saw each other so often, spent so much intimate, sweaty time together, it was almost as if we hadn't considered socializing outside the base. Leave it to Elle to be the one to remedy that.

Elle threw open the door as I raised my arm to show off the four-pack of peach Bartles & Jaymes I'd brought. Jean was coming up the path behind me, a slim brown bag in hand.

"Hey, ladies," Elle grinned. "Welcome to chez Elle and Macon."

"Nice place," I said. "I got lost three times."

"It's a new development," Elle replied. "Come on in."

Elle led us through the foyer, past the expansive living room, and through to the eat-in kitchen. "Would you mind organizing drinks while I finish setting up snacks and get the wine open?"

"Of course." I grabbed a wine cooler and put the other three in the fridge. "Jean? What'll it be?"

Jean walked over and peeked into the refrigerator. "I'll figure something out," she said. The rest of the women filtered in, and I was immediately struck by the smell of soap and perfume.

"We clean up good," I observed. Marion's hair was down and flowing now she was off duty, and I realized this was the first time I've seen some of them in jeans.

"It's weird that we're clean," Amanda said, tilting her nose in the air and sniffing.

We laughed, and Elle made sure everyone had drinks. Wine in hand, she beckoned. "Follow me."

She led us to the living-room, where the brand-new cream carpet was covered with a drop cloth, a ring of disembodied white T-shirts, a rainbow of decorative glue pens, and a blizzard's worth of glitter.

"What on God's green earth is this?" I asked. "You didn't tell us we were coming over for arts and crafts night."

Amanda had no such cynical reservations. "I love crafting! This is going to be great."

"Gather round the T-shirts," Elle said, "and let's make some history."

I sat in front a one-size-fits all shirt and checked out the tools I had to decorate it. Elle was right; this might actually be fun. I felt stress starting to leave my body as I surveyed the empty canvas.

"Clearly C-Group is the *best*—just kidding, Jean, I'm sure D-Group is great too—so why not make it official?" Elle explained. "I thought we could come up with a motto, put it on all our shirts, then decorate with our own flair."

"What's our motto going to be?" Amanda jumped in, staring at her shirt like she'd been commissioned to paint the king's portrait.

"I had some ideas," Elle said, a glint in her eye. "First of all, in the upper right corner, what about a logo like 'C: Where you wanna be'? I came up with that in the shower."

We all agreed. "Perfect," Nadine nodded. "Now we need something big for the main design."

I said, "I think it's obvious what our motto is."

"Yes," said Elle.

"Do *what*?" I called out.

They all yelled back, "Fuck *that*!"

All of them, that is, except Laurie.

I shot her a look. "Did you say '*fudge* that?'"

"I did," Laurie admitted. "I'm not a prude or anything. But when I was a kid, a camp counselor told me that word has a violent and anti-woman history, so I try to avoid it."

None of us could argue with that. I still intended to wear the obscenity on my shirt, but I planned to look up the meaning of it later.

"Gimme a pen." Marion was reaching out for some colored glue. "I'm in."

"Fair enough," Laurie acquiesced. "I'll just bleep out the U-C-K."

We began drawing and sprinkling glitter and laughing like schoolgirls.

"Can you pass the pink?" I asked Nadine.

She handed it over.

"*Nadine*," Elle said. "Your *arms*."

Everyone looked up. Nadine grinned and stretched her legs out, sitting perpendicular to the tarp. "It's crazy, right? Only a few weeks in. Check out these muscles." She crooked her bicep. "And you know what's funny? I never thought I *wanted* muscles. But now…now I feel *powerful*. Do you know what I mean?"

"I get it," Amanda said. "Stairs are nothing to me now. Grocery shopping feels different. It's the little things."

"And we get to kick ass for all those women in the military," Donna said. "No woman left behind."

Nadine raised her wine glass. "To strong women," she said.

I held my glass in the center. "To warriors like us."

Everyone clinked glasses.

"To warriors like us!" My friends echoed.

I instinctively felt—or convinced myself—that Marion understood we weren't trying to take away from what soldiers go through. We were trying to do our part the best way we could, and we were suffering for our goals, like anyone, and we needed to let off steam, like anyone. But I never would, and hoped I never did, try to compare our seven months to a soldier's service and sacrifices.

Elle refilled our drinks, and we finished our shirts and then made one for Eric, and at the end she reminded us, "Everyone wear your shirts on Monday! Let's show Eric what the best group is."

The next day, as promised, Elle bounded up to me as soon as I walked through the door. "Girl! You wore it! We all did...look."

Eric sauntered over. I grabbed my shirt's hem and stretched out the fabric for him to see. "That sums this group up perfectly," he said wryly, shaking his head. "Who's got a camera?"

I dashed out to my car and grabbed a disposable camera I always carried with me, and someone took a photo of our fronts and backs, all of us stacked on the squat machine, with Eric there, too, wearing the one we'd made for him, and that moment was frozen in time.

PART THREE

JAGGED LITTLE PILL

8

No one said it would be easy

Eric was the center of my Army universe, but A-Group trainer Chris Palmer was also quietly killing it every day. While I was still asleep every morning, those type-A machines were rising before sunrise to train with Chris, a young newlywed with a day job outside of the study. He stood before them in those first days and, unsmiling, told his test subjects what he expected. There was little chit-chat about personal lives in the beginning, and no joking around—most of them had to rush off to full-time jobs, school, or both when the session ended.

Their days started so early, in fact, that the A-Group women generally showed up with empty stomachs. As a horrified Mary replied once when I asked her about her breakfast habits, "I never ate *before*. Who works out with a full belly?" Fair point, though on the other hand I wasn't sure I could do an extreme 90 minutes with an empty tank.

If Eric eased his groups into the athlete's life with relaxed banter that served to calm and distract us from the pain, Chris started like a no-nonsense drill sergeant. His team lifted when told to, filed out silently to Cement Hill for their runs, and if they ever did complain, he was fine with it. "I took that to mean we were headed in the right direction," he told me.

Jane, who'd come off an extended stay on the couch to join up, was in A-Group with Mary and Veronica, a naturally muscular woman who would turn out to be a top performer. Jane was prepared for someone like Chris to greet her as she set foot on the base.

"I was like well, the study's run by guys; are they all gonna be alpha males? I wouldn't call it a fear, but it was an anxiety that I had," she confided in me. At first, Chris seemed to be as tough as she expected.

It didn't help that the nerves many of us had in the beginning were hard to shake, especially on tough tests like the VO2 max, Jane adds. "I remember being on the treadmill feeling like, what *is* this? How long am I going to be able to run, am I going to pass out? I'm drooling, this is embarrassing. I remember starting out with a mixture of anticipation and trepidation and a little anxiety and nervousness."

My trainer heard all about Chris's methods on an infuriatingly regular basis. "I was always getting feedback on Chris from some of the subjects," Eric told me. "He's the serious one. I'd been coaching for years, and after working as a fitness director at a health club, I was used to working with people and joking around."

Eric's most recent job involved instructing what he calls "ladies who lunch" in the gym at a country club, a world away from Ev and Pete's effort in the austere environs of the military, and he was also working at Fitchburg State and a part-time track coach.

Chris, on the other hand, had been focused on training college athletes to produce high-stakes wins. "I had just come from getting athletes to do what they were supposed to do coaching at UMass," said Chris, who worked closely with Brianna Scurry, the famed U.S. soccer goalie, and fellow players who made it to the Olympics. "We don't fuck around."

Eric heard about Chris's methods and assured me in one of our interviews that he would never "fuck around" either (I can attest to that), but adds, "You can make people work hard, but you don't have to be that asshole football coach who yells and screams at kids who are fifteen years old."

Chris agreed with that much. "Yeah, you shouldn't do that. I give them the time, attention, and motivation to perform to their best. They'll respect you if you respect them."

Early on in the study, it would remain to be seen whose, if anyone's, strategy would produce results. It would be a long road for the two men as they took civilian women with varying levels of skill, interest, fitness and motivation and tried to make them strong and survivable, as is the Army's unshakeable goal.

Eric's index finger hit relentlessly on the metal slider. *Tap. Tap. Tap.*

It was weigh-in day again, and I was ready for a significant loss. I'd been patient. Each week I stood on that scale, sore and tall and strong, arms at my sides, and every week I'd lose zero or one pounds when I'd been trying for five or ten. I was eating less junk and more real food. A bean burrito instead of frozen yogurt, a salad instead of a sandwich, one beer instead of two. Oddly, I'd become less hungry over those first weeks; the gnawing pangs I'd had since the extreme liquid diet the year before had abated as the excessive exercise began.

Our trainers didn't tell us how to eat. Nutrition wasn't a part of the study, though when people asked for tips, they would pass on a few ideas here and there. Some subjects with much less—or nothing—to lose were, annoyingly, aiming now for ripped abs, which meant I'd been subjected to the beginnings of the six-pack club, a handful of test-subjects who'd gotten strong and cocky and decided a rippled midriff was within reach.

I had to admit to a dollop of schadenfreude when Eric would shake his head and remind them repeatedly, *It's genetic. You melt away all the fat and see what's there. You'll have at six-pack or you won't. But sure, we can try.* Elle was one of the six-pack crew, and while I was supportive from afar, I stayed out of that conversation. I would never have a hard stomach, and therefore would not kill myself trying.

"One pound," Eric said that day, marking the number down.

"*One pound?* Fuck that," I snapped.

"Next," Eric said.

That young blond soldier was there again after the day's workout; he tended to be around whenever Marion was. They were chatting with Eric by the door, and I meant to get out of the room before they even knew I was there. The young private looked like every frat boy who'd ever stared past me like I wasn't there, and every boy in gym class who snickered as I stumbled. But, in trying to slip past them invisibly, I tripped on a piece of metal jutting out from one of the machines. "*OW!*"

The man, a boy, really, lunged out and caught me, righted me, and smiled shyly.

"You OK?"

"I'm good," I smiled back. I couldn't help it. He emanated gentleman-ness and spoke with a Southern twang. Billy was his name, and it turned out he was Marion's boyfriend.

Marion was watching my near-catastrophe with concern, but *she* wasn't smiling. Come to think of it, what I'd thought of as stoicism in the short time I'd known her was starting to seem like something else. I'd kept my weight worries mostly to myself so far, but I wasn't the only C-Group woman hiding a part of me. Others had secrets, too, and finally one day one of them couldn't help but reveal hers.

Later that week, it was a beautiful day on the banks of Lake Cochituate. The scent of cut grass was in the air, the sky was a blazing azure, and Elle was laughing as she often was. A young, preternaturally happy woman with a strong moral compass, Elle had become our social director. We'd gone dancing and drinking, sipped wine at her house, and began socializing mostly amongst ourselves because no one else could possibly understand what we were going through. With Elle's help, the shyer ones among us had opened up and grown closer. And so we couldn't help but notice Marion was quieter than normal. When she asked if someone would spot her on the bench press, I volunteered.

I stood over her. She lifted. She grunted. I cheered her on. She lifted again. She stopped, and I looked down to find out why.

Tears were pouring down her face. I moved to her side of the bench. "What's wrong? Hey, it's OK…OK." I said this despite not knowing whether it would be OK or not. "Tell me. What's *wrong*, Marion?"

Elle was over in a shot. This wasn't good—and it wasn't like Marion. Army girl wasn't a crier. Elle, Nadine and I surrounded Marion in the corner by the squat machine.

"What. Is. *Wrong*," I demanded again, because I knew if we could pinpoint her problem, we could get to work fixing it.

She laughed through tears. "I don't *know*," she said. "It's nothing."

"What do you mean it's nothing? It's not nothing!" Elle cried.

We were utterly confused, the three of us, her girlfriends, ones you'd call ride-or-die in new millennium-speak. We were going to be there for Marion no matter what was the matter.

Elle said, "You can tell us. We won't judge you."

Nadine was nodding along, and as she often did, she was listening more than talking. Cocking her head and squinting her eyes. She was a mom already, she'd been married, and she had thirty-three years under her belt to Marion's twenty.

And then, like someone turned off a faucet, Marion's tears stopped as quickly as they'd begun. She cleared her throat and pointed to the vertical machine. "I've got abs to do," she said.

"Uh uh," Elle shook her head.

"I'm OK," Marion assured us, smiled, walked over to the vertical/horizontal bench. "I promise."

Later, we did our Cement Hill run and I briefly forgot about Marion's moment. The tears had come out of nowhere and disappeared just as fast. A few days later, I was waiting to get on the upright rows machine and watched Marion lift for two sets before I realized she was silently weeping again.

"That's it," I said. "Tell us what's going on *right now*."

My mind was racing with possibilities. Problems with Billy? Her parents. Another boy. Her career? A mean drill instructor?

Elle joined us. "That's it," she echoed. "We're going to meet after training and talk this out."

But first it was back to Cement Hill, where Marion stayed ahead with no tears and Donna kept me sane. She was a no-nonsense kind of woman who continued to stick by me as I worked to run faster for longer. I asked her flat-out her why she never left me behind, and her answer was brutally, adorably honest: "Because you're the only one I can keep up with." She joined this thing, she told me, because she felt uncomfortably out of shape. She thought she was heavy and looked heavy. In my eyes she was the epitome of "normal," something I'd never been, and her confession surprised me.

"Aside from the fact we were doing something pretty important, the big draw to the study was to get in shape and lose some weight," she explained. "I've never considered myself to be fit. I've always looked at pictures of myself and go *hmmm*…I don't look like anybody who could do something like that." And yet she was, and she did. I viewed Donna as stoic and kind and capable. I didn't know at the time that she was keeping a secret of her own.

After our run that day, Elle and I ushered Marion to a quiet nook outside.

"I cry all the time," she told us through tears. "Sometimes I cry all day. I'm sad…all the time."

"You need to see a doctor," Elle said. "You can't go on like this."

"Is there someone on-base you can talk to?" I asked.

"I guess," she'd replied. It occurred to me a bit late that *we* were the people on base she could talk to. "I don't know what this is. I just want to go back to bed."

Elle and I exchanged glances. The fact was, Marion had no reason she could point to. It was 1995 and clinical depression was still a distant concept to many people. None of us standing there that day, including Marion, understood how a person could be going about her nice life and then suddenly get slammed by a tsunami of sadness, and when that pulls back for a bit, the person is left with agonizing depths of nothingness and an inability to care about anything. I'd had dark thoughts and had been wracked with sobs of desperation and grief myself (mostly in my teen years), but the breakdowns were generally situational. There was a trigger. A *reason*. On good days, I felt OK. When nice things happened, I was happy.

Finally, Elle ordered, "Make an appointment to see the doctor today. You promise?"

"I promise." Marion, our tough, happy-go-lucky friend, replied.

With more than forty women spread over four groups, it was inevitable each unit would develop its own personality. With a stern trainer and no time to spare, A-Groupers became known for their competitive nature and, I'm loathe to say it, excellent results. Veronica was a machine. Mary was turning into a finely tuned athlete. Jane was improving faster than almost anyone. Every group had their winners, though individual performance wasn't a focus of the study.

B-Group trained too late in the morning for anyone with a nine-to-five job to join, and their members were a bit of a mish-mash. Eric said they reminded him fondly of the "ladies who lunch" back at his previous job, though these were no country club princesses. They tore it up as much as anyone, and to keep things interesting B-Group's volunteers prided themselves on the nicknames they assigned each other. Denise LePage, who lived in Natick not far from the base, was "Chopper."

"Spider" was a take-no-shit blonde with a big job and one particular goal that didn't necessarily mesh with the study's purpose—she wanted to lose weight. Lots of it. The scientists would rather she eat plenty and get strong. "Bruiser" drove down every day from the North Shore, and, says Denise, "she could lift like 80,000 pounds a hundred times and we're like, uh, we're not gonna beat that. I was Chopper because I have this 1975 bike I ride to the base."

Denise kept showing up because of the camaraderie, but she'd started this thing to make a point. "I grew up in the seventies when girls were smacked down: 'Oh, you can't do this, only boys can do that.' *I'll* tell you what I can and can't do," she told me. "When this came up I was like, I totally have to do this. We can do the same things as men, you know what I'm sayin'? All of us in the study had something to prove. Just because we're female doesn't mean we can't do anything a guy can do. And we're all there to prove it."

B-Group had some top performers, too, including Lina, to name one. Another subject happened to have the same last name as Boston's longest-serving mayor who remained in office for nearly two decades until his death in 2014. "I nicknamed Stacey Meninno 'The Mayor,'" Eric laughed during one of our interviews. "Every weekend I come home and the news will be talking about Mayor Menino, and every morning I'm dealing with Stacey, so she became The Mayor."

B-Group's Mayor was a doer. Legend has it she

implemented policy swiftly and decisively, plotting a secret shortcut through the running route I dreaded so much. B-Group would use the device sparingly, I'm told, saving it for days when they were truly exhausted. Eric discovered the subterfuge before long, and let them get away with it for the most part because, he said, they were working hard otherwise and took The Mayor's Route only occasionally. "When it was time to run, they used to whisper amongst each other: 'are we gonna run the whole thing, or are we taking the Mayor's Route?'" Eric relayed to me.

C-Group was made up of the meanderers. We'd stroll in for a mid-day workout and then wander out when it was over, sometimes after a post-workout chat and a laugh, depending on babysitters and deadlines and nap schedules and client meetings (for the women *and* the kids); there wasn't a nine-to-fiver among us. Our group was smaller, more diverse, and possibly a bit older on average. We were the best by every measure, obviously.

The after-work crowd in D-Group reported being more businesslike in the beginning, though that focus brought them together in their own way. Their take-no-prisoners grit begat a quieter connection, a tacit pact to keep their heads down, do the work and keep pushing. Stacey Coady, a law student, was one of the strongest women—if not *the* strongest—in the study. She could lift *244 pounds* to thirty inches. She'd recently given up her apartment in Boston's North End and moved to the suburbs with a new boyfriend, so was stuck riding her bicycle every day from Wellesley to law school in Boston both ways. "It wasn't a quest for fitness—it was because I didn't have a car," she told me, half-laughing at the absurdity of it.

She and I had at least one thing in common. "Even being an athlete in three sports in high school, I never liked running," Stacey says. "The base being on the water is helpful for me. There are parts of it that are scenic and that helps me forget."

D-Group turned out to be the way Stacey, a pretty, statuesque woman with dark-blonde hair, could finally embrace the trait she was most conflicted about. "I don't know how or why I was born strong," Stacey told me. "It wasn't something I worked toward. Some of my sisters are petite size fours or fives, and I'm almost six feet tall and got the big bones and the strong back."

But once she joined the study, "I felt validated. I had always struggled with my strength and was embarrassed by it a lot of times, like when someone would be moving an air conditioner out of the windows at home or work. Other people are like, 'oh let's go get three more people to do this' and I'm like, 'can you just look the other way for a minute?' I could do it myself easily. I've since turned that around and flipped the switch, and am not ashamed of it. I try to be proud."

Back to A-Group, the only one trained by Chris Palmer. There was a twist ending to Chris's brusque beginnings: The guy, it turned out, is a big softie, something his charges discovered before too long.

"I was nervous about how tough he was," Jane said. "And then I got to know Chris and saw he's super nice.

He's always there for us. I was really relieved about that."

Mary echoes Jane's words about that side of him, crediting Chris for helping bring out the fighter in her. "I always found him to be tough but kind, funny, a good listener, and genuinely a good person. You wanted to be more like him."

I wasn't in his group, but I'm with them—I always found him a generous spirit, an excellent listener and an articulate speaker. With all this adoration sent Chris's way, Eric began to grow weary of the glowing reviews his counterpart was receiving.

"Chris was a little more serious with everyone, but then he started getting into the training and everybody started loving Chris. I started hearing, 'Chris is better looking than you.' 'He's fifteen years younger than you.' I'm like yeah, I know, so what."

"Basically the point is it took a little while for A-Group to warm up to me," Chris said.

"I usually *start* like that," Eric hit back.

I laughed myself to tears watching their banter. It was all OK, anyway; a little friendly competition never hurt anyone.

Catherine: 2015

Catherine Afton was gearing up for Officer Candidates School (OCS), a six-week course meant to weed out the candidates who can't hack it as a Marine. There are load-bearing hikes, sleep deprivation, and a shit-ton of yelling.

Rumors, legends and tips for how to survive those six weeks filter down through generations of Marines.

"I was so hyped up for three years, every Monday at six a.m. I had a class about OCS," Catherine says. "I was constantly being told how hard it was and I had been on so many fitness plans, I was making sure nothing that could've been in my control would be a problem once I got there. I was hiking up and down the streets around school just to practice, so I didn't step out of line."

The summer after her junior year, Catherine packed her things and made the trip to Quantico, where she was assigned to train in a group of 35 women. She was right to worry about "stepping out of line." If you stumble, fall or can't keep up on those marches, you face humiliation and possible disciplinary action. If you lag enough times, it can get you kicked out. The course is physically tough—but by design, it's also a very deliberate test of mental strength.

"The first hike was three miles, and everyone's trying to prove themselves," Catherine remembers. "My platoon commander is there to teach us what an officer should be like. We were told, 'everyone behind that tree is considered falling out.' *So* few people stayed in. I fell out of that. Once you've fallen out of something, it's hard; I always empathize with people who do. Some fall out every single time—it's mental. One of my best friends is five feet even, and she stayed up. The pack is bigger than her. She passed."

Some say there's no better test of mental strength at OCS than the Quigley. As one person familiar with the Quigley reported cryptically, "they thicken it in all sorts of ways."

Another person I spoke to was happily specific: "People pee in it. That's a thing." It was designed in 1977 by men for men, meant to replicate the conditions in the jungles of Vietnam with their hidden booby traps and impossible obstacles. As an article in the Marine Corps Base Quantico's publication marking the fiftieth anniversary of the course explained in 2017, "The assignment given to then-1st Lt. William J. Quigley was simple and to the point. Create a course where 'each candidate should look like they tangled with two constipated pit bulls, and lost.'"

In a letter read out at the anniversary celebration, Quigley wrote that bestselling author Tom Clancy once proclaimed that "the mind that conceived this thing had to have been demented," according to the article.

Catherine would be struggling through the sludge that summer, but before she could show her mettle, she found herself in an unnerving predicament. She woke up one morning, looked in the mirror, and saw a creeping rash on her face. She ignored it and went about her business; she knew that falling out in any sense of the word risked her place there, her rank, her ROTC scholarship. Catherine pretended it wasn't happening and continued training; she didn't want to give her superiors any reason to single her out.

"I did take a lot of yelling there," she remembers. "I was so bad at drill. For my life I could not do it; I was one off when marching with a rifle. I never stopped, though. I just took it and kept on going. In a way it was comforting, because I knew I was saving other people from getting yelled at. I was a fun person to yell at."

And so she remained in denial even as the raised rash grew worse. "I was supposed to be out in front of the line leading, and I had all this stuff all over my face," she recalls with a groan. "It was yellow and crusty and random instructors would run by and say, 'What the fuck's all over your face, candidate?'"

Finally, it became clear she had to be seen by a medic. "I told the doctor I *really* don't think it's herpes, but he gave me herpes medication. So I took it every night but it didn't get better, and they're like, 'oh wait, that's not it,' so they sent me to another doctor who said, 'you have impetigo, which is very common in five-year-old boys.' That was sweet," she adds wryly of the highly contagious skin infection. "It was so much fun. I was the first at OCS to get it."

The fun was just beginning, though. Catherine found herself one steamy summer day, in full uniform, ready to sink into the Quigley's brown muck. Barbed wire stretched over rolling wet logs the candidates were expected to maneuver through while holding fast to their weapons. "Some of the girls were terrified of water," Catherine recalls, noting she couldn't speak for the men because her group did not generally train with males. "Fellow candidates were afraid of getting into this muck."

But get in they did, and as their team muscled through while an officer hovered over them shouting anything but encouragement, one woman could barely function. She was slow, scared, falling behind. Catherine wasn't doing much better, she says now, especially as she faced the most frightening part for many who endure it: The culverts. The concrete tubes are the things of nightmares even for those *without* a bad case of claustrophobia, because they were submerged beneath the goo and each person had to make it through holding her weapon and praying for breath.

The yelling was relentless. And Catherine, always in the top few through her young life, always putting mind over matter, was doing terribly.

"We were actually really far behind, and the person we were with was constantly yelling that we were the worst group he had ever seen."

Ha, I said. *WERE you the worst, though? Not really?*

"No, I think we were," she nodded. "We were pretty bad. Everyone around us was telling us that too. People were laughing at us. The girl who was struggling most was getting yelled at, and we couldn't go back or cheer her on. That's one of the things they tell you—'stop cheering. We're not cheerleaders here.' We had to sit there, we weren't allowed to go back to cheer them on, and we don't have watches. We have no sense of time."

OCS proved to be as tough as they say, and it was the smallest and most basic things that kept them going, like friendship, stationery and cough drops. "The *cough drops*," Catherine remembers as if they were truffles at a Michelin-starred restaurant. "Everyone liked cough drops. At OCS you weren't allowed to have your own candy or food but we could get cough drops...we'd get whatever kind they sold, green, fruity green *cough drops*."

Aside from small comforts, it was the pain that cleaved them together for the duration. "The way you can get closest is through suffering," Catherine says. "OCS was tough, but going through hard times brings people closer. What made it so phenomenal was everyone helping each other. I wouldn't have graduated if I didn't have the girls beside me to do little things to make sure I didn't mess up and to help with things I didn't do on my own."

She responded in kind. "Whatever I could give back I would try to do," she says. "We're all facing this external force we can't control, but we *can* control how we're going to react to it. I thought that was so beautiful. I realized then this career was right for me. I value emotional toughness in spite of physical or mental pain. That's what the Marine Corps prides itself on."

She recalls that through her experience working to become a Marine, only a few areas were gender-normed. Some of the runs, for example, and, "When I first started, I couldn't do pullups. I *thought* I couldn't do it, but I rose to the occasion. If you have to do it, a lot of times, you can."

There was, she says, an odd feeling of loss when the acute pain of the course finally abated. "At the end of OCS, the person who yelled at me the most called me into her office and we had a semi-civil encounter. She was yelling at me while also asking me where I was from, getting to know me without breaking the barrier of her being a disciplinarian.

"The night before I graduated I couldn't sleep. I knew I was going to have to leave all these girls. I realized there was no way I could've graduated without all of them. You don't have your phone at OCS, but you can write letters. They gave us a lot of stationery, so I wrote a letter to every girl in the platoon thanking them. Going through that was a wonderful exercise; you don't do anything alone. Some make the argument we shouldn't be separate," Catherine posits. "But I like the girls together—putting us altogether worked well. I think the moment I felt like I actually belonged [in the Marines] was at OCS."

That year was, as it happened, also the first time in the history of this country that a woman could pursue whatever military path she wanted. Whatever section of the Marine Corps Catherine had an aptitude for, a desire to engage in, was open to her in a way it never had been to women before. Catherine graduated OCS and was now a Second Lieutenant in the United States Marine Corps. But she wasn't done proving herself—a longer and more painful trial to show the Corps what she was made of awaited her.

June 1995

I wasn't in the mood for O'Hara's attitude the next weigh-in day. I pulled up to the booth and he made eye contact right away, nodded, and waved me on. Extraordinary. He wasn't technically *friendly*, but he was bordering on attentive and alert, which was new. I was past caring. I was heading for the scale, and I'd prepared by reducing my calories over the week and then, when the weekend hit, I'd allowed myself a slice of pizza or three with the gang from the paper after a night out, plus a couple of light beers and a tumbler of Purplesaurus Rex, a favorite cheap drink of the Broke New Adult (recipe: A few sprinkles of Purplesaurus Rex-flavor Kool-Aid; cheap-ass vodka from a plastic bottle; lots of ice). Oh, and did I mention I worked out for eight hours with an Olympic-trials-caliber trainer?

I burst into the training room that day and stormed that scale. *Tap, tap, tap* went Eric's finger. "Same as last week." He said it with his usual flat shrug followed by a wiggle of his fingers signaling the next victim to step up.

I stormed back off the scale and took a walk to the back of the room.

"What?" Asked Horace the intern, half laughing at my drama.

"Is it against the law to murder a scale?"

"I don't think so. Stop worrying about it. You're getting fit. That's the important thing," Horace claimed irrelevantly. I gave him the evil eye.

"You don't want to be like Beatrice," he ill-advisedly continued.

"Why not?" I was pretty sure I'd met her briefly—she was that pretty blonde with a big job.

"Have you seen her? She's lost a ton of weight since this started."

I didn't bother to ask why I *wouldn't* want to be Beatrice. All I wanted right that minute was to *be* Beatrice. *That's it*, I thought. No more messing around.

I got on with it, and a few days later Marion took Elle and me aside after training and gave us the update: She'd gone to see the base doctor, and there was hope that Marion's melancholy could be managed or even banished. "The Army doctor sent me to see a psychiatrist, and I cried the entire visit," she told us. He put her on an anti-depressant, and she was taking it as ordered.

The medicine started to do its job, but we kept a keen eye on our young friend. We needed her.

9

I'll be there for you

I cried laughing every week with Eric. He could roll his eyes at me and I'd crack up; he could call me out on my *I can'ts* and get me to do the last five sit-ups from across the room. I knew he was a diversion, but there was no denying I was growing attached. I was melting under the heat of his focus on me. He'd turned his eyes on every one of his subjects and wouldn't look away until he was done with us. Still, I wasn't *entirely* stuck on him. There was a guy in ad sales at the paper I had my eye on. With a sweep of brown hair and milk chocolate eyes, he was *sooo beautiful,* as I wrote in my diary. In a display of creative brilliance I dubbed him Advertising Guy. Before long, things started heating up: He now always made eye contact and held it whenever I passed him in the hall. And then, one day, when he was inexplicably walking through the newsroom, we crossed paths, and when he said *Hi* to me I proceeded to trip over a garbage can, and then I ran away.

And there was Ford, of course, who I'd neglected badly, secretly hoping he'd give up on me. One Friday night the gang from the paper went on a bar crawl in the general Marlborough/Hopkinton/Ashland area. I was young, free and single and I had a designated driver. I drank beer and then turned to vodka cranberries. When I saw Ford in a corner with a couple of pals, I was over there like a shot, and hid nothing of my irritation. He saw me across the room and met me halfway.

"Hi," I said. "What a coincidence."

"There are literally two bars in town. It's not that coincidental."

He smiled, I smiled. "I haven't seen you in awhile. How's the Army?"

I showed him some bruises, and he couldn't see a thing in the low light but congratulated me nonetheless, and just as I was about to say I had to get back to my friends, he said, "I better get back to my friends. By the way, do you still want to see *Batman*? How about next week?"

"Sure," I said.

"He's cute," Rebecca said when I left him. "Why didn't I know about him?"

"There's nothing to know." She let it go, and I bought her a drink. It was

good to see her out and about. I was out of the office for hours every day now, and she was running around covering schools *and* cops, and I'd been missing her.

Monday in the gym, Elle asked me for a Ford update

and I gave her a vague response because I was feeling vague about him. As she did her incline sit-ups, she said, "It's time you figured this out." *Inhale.* "We'll do a barbecue this weekend at my house." *Breathe, grunt.* "I'll ask Marion and Billy to come, too. We'll make it a triple date."

I put in the call to Ford's answering machine, and the next day he informed my voicemail that he'd attend, but would drive himself there from the gym. He pulled up outside Elle's as I was getting out of my car. He didn't come over, so I took a step toward her front door. Ford stood by his car with his arms hanging awkwardly by his sides.

"You ready?" I asked. "You'll love my new friends. They're really fun."

He regarded me for a long moment. "Let's not do this."

"I promised them I would…" I looked at him closer, standing there in his Levis, slightly sagging on his thin frame, in a Polo shirt and sun-streaked hair in the front from being on his dad's boat. "Oh." It took me a second, but I got it. He looked slightly embarrassed, nervous, and a little bit like he felt sorry for me, which I hate. "Really?"

"We both know. Don't we? If it's going nowhere, we shouldn't keep doing this."

"This." Ouch. But also, *Yay.* I felt bad; I knew I'd hurt him, but I also felt a *thud* of rejection with his words. And then, oddly, I felt as if the weight of a backpack was lifted off my shoulders. Ford Simmons had the rare maturity and guts to say it. He didn't ghost me, he didn't fade out, he didn't disappear. He'd been the brave one.

I went inside and told them what happened. I made

them all promise not to pity me, and after a few beers we all forgot about it. Elle's adorable children were a buffer, as was the food, the grill, and the guests. Macon and Elle were both excellent hosts and she was smiling and laughing as usual around her husband, but not so much *with* him, and I noted that didn't fit with the picture of bliss she'd painted on that first walk back in May.

Summer kept on top of us with a thick layer of humidity and a tireless chorus of insects buzzing around the woods and the lake, but we never let up. I wrote another front-page feature that ran with a photo of Nadine squatting a hundred pounds, pink bow tied at the top holding her curls back, a purple tank-top and fingerless gloves, with *Show of strength* emblazoned beneath her badass sneer. There was a quote from Pete talking about support for us on the base, which conflicted with my experiences of disdain directed our way. Like so many things we believe we are seeing in sharp relief, there is always gray in the spaces between; both things were quite possibly true. Some were rooting for us, and some were getting out the popcorn ready to watch us fail. Just like every other place you'll ever be in life.

In any case, we were getting used to being recognized outside the base as our stories of pain, triumph and hope captured the interest of our corner of Massachusetts. More than one delivery driver stopped his truck to throw me support, with one tooting his horn and calling out, "You all are amazing. Keep it up!" A mail carrier caught Elle on her way out to the mailbox in her robe one morning and shouted, "Tell the girls we're rooting for you all down at the post office!" And Elle would make a muscle for him before running back inside to her kids.

The outside world hadn't forgotten we were there, but the Army was keeping the media at bay. Rumors of network TV and celebrity journalists like Diane Sawyer and big-city newspapers all clamoring to see what we were up to persisted, which raised my hackles; this was *my* baby now. *Let the underdogs run with it,* I thought. To my great joy, the Army did.

Summer was the season of the mother in C-Group. I was fairly certain ours was the only training group with Romper Room happening alongside our sandbag drags. Everett and Eric blinked nervously when kids turned up unannounced and without apology. Laurie brought her young daughters to the base along with a babysitter, Nadine brought her three-year-old daughter and a minder once or twice, and Elle brought her girls a bunch of times that summer in a crisp, *Here we are!* kind of way. She simply appeared with two little tow-heads and a teenager to watch them. Because Elle and I were growing so close, I'd already gotten to know her girls, ages three and five. One day when we were racing around the base, when we hit the quiet side along the banks of the lake, little bespectacled, curious Mona burst out and ran alongside us.

"Run, mommy! Run!"

"Sara, look! I'm running with you!"

She had the sweet voice of an angel, and she reminded me why we were doing this. This *mattered.* This girl would be a woman one day, and she deserved every opportunity to use the gifts she was given, whatever she'd discover them to be as she grew. Elle reached out and took Mona's hand. "Run with me now," she said. "Come on. We'll finish together." We all, eight women and two little girls, ran toward the future with bright eyes and a fire in our bellies.

On another day, Laurie's girls watched as we struggled under a blazing sun. Laurie would fan herself on the hottest days and shake her head. "This heat is off the charts. Sometimes I wish I was in the early morning group."

"You're doing great," Elle said, slapping her on the back.

"I'm just a regular person. Some of you are natural athletes, but I'm a regular person doing this, and don't you think this is *unbelievably* hard?"

"I do," I said, raising one hand and wiping my brow with the other.

As it happened one especially sizzling day, Laurie's daughters were taking a keen interest in us. They were terribly worried about their mom as she gasped and limped along on one of our runs, and soon the upsetting vision became too much for little Jasmine. The nine-year-old sprang up and ran to Laurie, who stopped for a moment to explain she mustn't be disturbed until her workout was over. Before she obeyed, Jasmine held out one little fist and revealed a handful of well-worn Goldfish crackers.

"Here, mommy," she said. "They'll make you better."

Laurie's heart swelled with the offer. She popped one in her mouth and sent Jasmine away, assuring the girl she was

OK. She kept running that day, heartened that her

children would see how hard she was working. Now that she'd walked the walk, hiked the hike, and run the run, she could ask the same of them, she told me in one chat, "without feeling like a hypocrite. That's really, really cool."

So, yes—we were hot that summer. But we were never in danger from extreme weather. With human test subjects in their care and strict ethics rules governing their work, Everett and his team didn't mess around. They consulted Dr. Richard Gonzalez and Leander Stroschein of the Biophysics and Biomedical Modelling Division of the U.S. Army Research Institute of Environmental Medicine, who provided a heat-strain model to ensure conditions were safe for us. They used a contraption that measured "wet bulb globe temperature," which translates to the difficulty of keeping body temperature from rising during hard work, and what they came up with boiled down to this: We were damn hot, but we were never *scientifically* hot enough to call off a single day of training. Plus, we had Eric's special military grade equipment to cool us down: He'd whip out the garden hose and spray us as we ran past him at the base of Cement Hill. The team was never far from us with cups of cool water.

The same careful consideration was applied to the flipside of New England's intense seasons. During the colder months, Everett sought the help of Dr. Murray P. Hamlet, the authority on cold injury at the U.S. Army Research Institute of Environmental Medicine at the time, who set a lower limit of -2°C (28°F) for us to be asked to lug our backpacks outside. As with summer, the weather in the autumn of 1995 was never deemed cold enough for us to miss a session. There was one day not long before final testing when we got a call telling us not to bother coming in because of snow, not temperature; a blizzard hit and they decided to spare us the trip.

I was hungry again. I'd started obsessing and depriving, and I was jittery from too many meals replaced with cans of Slim-Fast, but I still looked the same. One day after my last infuriating weigh-in I tromped into the newsroom in my clunky hiking boots, baggy clothes, hair disheveled, probably stinking up the place. I had a story due by five and no time to shower after my workout.

I headed to my desk and passed the pod where my alleged good friend Blake sat. He shook his head, laughed, and proclaimed loudly as I walked by, "Whatever you do, don't shower on our account."

"I won't. But thanks for pointing out my questionable hygiene to the entire newsroom."

"I don't think there's anything questionable about it."

"Ha, ha."

"Man," Blake said, giving me one more quick once-over while laughing his deep belly laugh that rang through the room, "if I was working out as much as you are, I'd be wasting away."

I froze. His words were loud and blunt and embarrassing. And so, so true. This was something I was used to from men, the commenting on and the presumed ownership of my body: *Ooh, you're a big girl, aren't you? Looking good—keep it up! You've lost weight. If you just lost fifteen pounds you'd be hot…*

"Thank you," I replied at equal volume.

Blake's words were hurtful, and to say them so publicly—to say them at all—was thoughtless, but they weren't incorrect. It *was* harder for me to drop fat than other people, especially men. My body craved more and hoarded too efficiently after so much yo-yoing so young. My brain was wired differently, my metabolism was mean and sluggish after extreme dieting, and I was tired of apologizing for it. Calories in/calories out was a delightfully reductive refrain aimed at us our whole lives, but its major flaw is that if you're burning a fuck-ton fewer calories than the imprecise medical calculations said you should be, and your body told you that you needed more all the time, you'll almost always be taking in too many, because your math will always be wrong.

In a nice bit of timing, the next day I found my fight song. I was driving the old Celica down Rt. 30 when a woman's voice made me reach down and turn up the radio. It would've been WBCN that played it. "You Oughta Know" was released that July, and I took to it in a hot minute.

The feral scream in it was what got so many of us, making us feel a certain *way* when we heard it. Alanis Morissette and her primal call roared through my car radio that day and burrowed into my brain. It was scandalous with its talk of blowjobs in the theater and it was made for the young, and I sang it constantly, especially while pumping a hundred pounds of iron. I didn't turn the music down when I pulled up to O'Hara, who'd been nicer to me lately. And by nice, I mean he didn't view me with the usual combination of boredom and suspicion.

Eric barely looked up from his clipboard as I stepped onto the scale, or when he was tapping that balance with excruciating care, and as usual, I didn't look. Eric quit tapping. I stepped off and turned away.

"Down three," he said.

I turned back. "What?"

"Three. Pounds." He said it without inflection. No *good job*, no smile, no encouragement. I stood for a moment and took that in. No *Atta girl*, no *See? It's working! You'll be thin enough before you know it.* It was utterly refreshing. No one had ever *not* placed a value judgment on my weight before. Gaining was bad, a mark of shame; losing was *good*, to be celebrated and congratulated. Yet no one in this room was celebrating my weight loss, just as no one hassled me about being a squeak away from 200 pounds.

Extraordinary.

Later that day, Elle spotted me on the bench press. I could barely finish seven reps of the same weight I'd been lifting for two weeks.

"We all have our bad days," Elle assured me. "Keep trying."

Eric walked by on his way to help someone else and snapped, "That's what happens when you starve yourself."

I used my abdominal muscles, newly strong though still well hidden, to sit up.

"I didn't starve myself. I'm nowhere near losing like Beatrice is."

Eric stopped, turned, and said, "And we're not happy when that kind of weight loss affects your lifting. Do the work to be an athlete. The appearance stuff will happen." He moved on.

The appearance stuff. In three words he'd sidelined looks and zoomed in on performance. It was brand new, this dismissing of my jeans size or how I measured up under the male gaze. On my way out that day, Everett was getting ready for his own workout and looked up as I passed. He saw more than he let on, and understood more than he would say. "We don't want you hungry. We want you strong. I don't care what your weight is," he said, pointing to the scale. "I care how much weight you can *lift.*"

That was the day, the hour, the minute, and the second I let it go. My body was strong. It belonged to me. I wasn't ever going to give up my power and my peace to a scale again. The weight of that burden I'd carried for so long floated away. It didn't fit there; there was no space in that room for any of it.

Enough now.

Marion had stopped crying, and she told us she'd found out what Billy—so young and barely out of his teen years—was made of while she waited for the medicine to work.

"I don't think he understands exactly what I was going through, but he seems fine about it," Marion told me. "That's a lot to put on somebody and on a relationship, but he never seems annoyed or mad."

While Marion was opening up, Elle still avoided any talk of her marriage, despite her dreamy chatter on that first backpack walk. Macon had been conspicuously absent from some of our gatherings at her house, with work always the proffered excuse. When we were alone outside stretching one day, I asked her, "Are you two OK?"

"It's all fine," she assured me. "We don't get much time together. Work the kids, the study. All of it."

"Tell you what," I said. "I'll take the girls to the movies Sunday. Give you the day."

The next weekend, Elle strapped her girls in the backseat of their minivan and I drove us to see *Pocahontas*. I expected my friend to have raging sex, rattle the chandeliers, shake the house, and greet me at the door sweaty and disheveled. When I returned, Elle and Macon were cross-legged on the living-room floor organizing the last of their moving boxes. I was shocked—and annoyed. I didn't give up my precious weekend so my friend could *clean*. I didn't know then about marriage and how two people can live in the same house and still be far apart, and perhaps this was their only chance of getting close again in the quiet.

The shaming of Shannon Faulkner

That summer, a thousand miles away under the same sun, another civilian woman was stepping bravely onto military ground. Unlike me, she did it alone. Unlike my male leaders, hers were invested in her failure.

On August 12, 1995, twenty-year-old Shannon Faulkner became the first woman in the history of The Citadel military college to join its corps of cadets. By the time Shannon fell in line as the only female marching with the men at the traditionally all-male school, she was already exhausted after a years-long legal battle. Two years before, in 1993, a hopeful, brave eighteen-year-old Shannon had applied to the school (full name The Citadel, the Military College of South Carolina) hoping to discover if a career in military service was for her or not. She left her pronouns off her transcripts, and the public institution, assuming this Shannon on the application before them was male, admitted her. But when they realized their mistake, they whipped the acceptance away. Shannon refused to accept that kind of blatant discrimination and sued the school—which receives public funding—in 1993, asserting that its all-male student body was unconstitutional.

What followed was a relentless legal battle and campaign of harassment that drained Shannon and her family. Along with the school, locals, students and alumni added to the chorus of reasons to keep her out, most of them antiquated even for the time; the public college was holding fast to "tradition," falling back on "because it's always been that way," and, said one nineties-era cadet, "Women would inhibit discussions" in the classroom.

After a series of false starts, judicial orders, victories and stays, Shannon was allowed in January of 1994 to register at The Citadel as a day student living off campus, but could *not* participate in military training. By that summer, though, a judge ruled she *could* join the corps of cadets after all. The court also ordered Shannon to shave her head, just as the male cadets did.

"We literally had to battle everything," Shannon told me recently. "Every issue was us battling it or the other side battling it. Every little thing ended up being a court issue. Public opinion was, if they have to shave my head, that's fine—it's hair, it'll grow back. But I was a teenage girl, and in private I was like, 'they're gonna shave my *head*? They're gonna try to take back anything they can from me.'"

It turned out to be a moot point for the moment, because The Citadel quickly appealed the decision to let her become a full student. Still, Shannon refused to give up even as she was being put down, yelled at and demeaned in ways the average male cadet never would be. During her years-long court battle, T-shirts reading "1,952 bulldogs and one bitch" went on sale in Charleston. "Die Shannon" reportedly was scrawled on a nearby water tower, and someone commissioned "Shave Shannon" bumper stickers. The Citadel school newspaper dubbed her "Shrew Shannon" and cadets called her "Mrs. Doubtgender." The teenager became public property, a target and a punching bag. She grew so accustomed to the ugly treatment that she actually *thanked* a man once for menacing her on campus.

"I remember one cadet, after something had happened in the press, came up to me and said, 'I don't want you here,'" Shannon recalls. "I was like, 'That's OK. You know what? I want to thank you.' He said, '*why*?' 'Because you said it to my face. I don't care if you like me or if you want me here. The fact you'll say that to me so we can have a discussion, I'm OK with that.' He was like, 'everybody else is scared you're going to tell everyone we were rude to you.' Uh uh—nope. I never complained about someone saying it to my face. Claiming to be gentlemen and then calling me nasty names from the shadows? Making threats or anonymous comments in the school newspaper? That's cowardly. You saying it to my face, I can deal with."

Shannon and her lawyers kept pushing. She wanted to study to become a teacher, but entering The Citadel, she told me, was also meant to be a way to get a flavor for military life. The school kept fighting her until the bitter end, finally asking the Supreme Court to intervene to keep her out. When the court refused, Shannon moved into her barracks on Saturday, Aug. 12, carrying a flute case and sheet music. That Monday she donned her uniform at the start of Hell Week. Before she could experience the full brutal treatment of those first days, she developed stomach trouble and exhaustion from stress and training in 100-degree heat and was taken to the infirmary along with three other cadets. She later went to the hospital. When they finally cleared her to return to school, she decided not to go back.

On August 19, Shannon Faulkner dropped out of The Citadel. As thunder cracked overhead and rain poured down, a choked-up young fighter announced her decision to leave. Cheers rang out on campus when the news was blasted over the public address system. Shannon's own attorney admitted to some concern about how her dropping out would affect the bigger case going forward, but admitted, "I'm not the one who has to sleep alone in the barracks."

Shannon said her farewells with her head held high. "I was handling the corps," she said at the conference by way of explanation. "At this point in time the past 2 1/2 years came crashing down on me in an instant." She added, "I don't think there is any dishonor in leaving."

Twenty-five years later, she told me, "Nobody ever saw me cry until that very last day. Luckily it was raining. I promised myself they would never make me cry in public."

It looked to outsiders like she gave up before she even began. But *her* fight had been a prolonged one and it was now over. She'd changed the institution, and in some ways her country, forever. "I did it not just for me, but for the next woman," she says.

The day she dropped out, as she disguised tears in that rainstorm, my editors asked me to pick a side and write a column. No one made any suggestion about what I should write; they sent me off with an assignment and trusted I'd be wise. I wrote an opinion piece fueled by excitement and blister pain and all I'd suffered on those hot days without a thought to dropping out. There is nothing like the hubris of youth possessed by those know-it-alls with smooth skin and bright, unlined eyes, the lucky ones among us having seen nothing of real hardship and stuck in our own experience like it's the only show in town. There was no Internet to speak of, and I knew Shannon would never see my words.

The headline was “Faulkner failing all women.” I set the story up with sympathy, acknowledging in my lede that she’d taken on a tough role: “Shannon Faulkner has a lot stacked against her,” I generously allowed. A few lines like that later came the *buts*. Even though she’d suffered intense heat and relentless resistance and abuse, I proclaimed, “Her failing was in her arrogance.”

I went on, “Obviously she didn’t spend much time at all in the gym or at the track” before stepping onto the campus, said I, the woman who complained every day about lightly jogging up a short steep hill, and was no fitness model myself. I proceeded to scold her for giving up. She was one of *thirty cadets* to drop out that week, but Shannon—the woman who’d had to fight in ways the others couldn’t comprehend—was the only one pummeled for it, and would be for years to come. After my column ran, the local Boston ABC TV station set up an interview with me for the evening news. I am beyond grateful to this day they ended up cancelling. Within a day or so, I was hit with a freight train of regret and disgust at what I’d written. I considered asking editors if I could write a retraction to my own piece, but in the end I left it alone.

Nearly two decades later, in a 2012 interview with the *Post and Courier* newspaper, Shannon revealed why she left so abruptly: Someone who was on campus when she arrived threatened to kill her parents. What I didn’t know in 1995—what none of us prehistoric keyboard warriors bothered to understand—was that Shannon was already spent when she set foot at The Citadel. I didn’t dig deeper, and I didn't focus enough on the difference between Eric and his calls of support lifting me up as I ran and the cruel, angry people holding Shannon down as she tried to get her feet off the ground. Shannon Faulkner was cancelled before cancel culture existed.

When we got to talking after she agreed to be interviewed for this book, she graciously allowed me to apologize to her. I told her of my vile behavior and I hoped I wouldn't have done it if there was a chance she'd have seen what I wrote. I shuddered to think what it would've been like for her if Twitter had existed then.

Shannon replied, "I appreciate the apology. You were young. You didn't know any better. I don't know how I would have survived if there had been social media. I can't imagine how bad it would've gotten. There were all the opinion pages and hurtful [words] and none of them knew me. If people only knew, would they still say the same thing if this was your daughter or your sister doing this? Would you say the same things to her?"

I hope not, I told her, then asked how she dealt with the constant pressure and negativity around her. "In a lot of ways I didn't," she says. "I dealt with things by not dealing with it. That ended up being part of my downfall. I internalized all of it. I was actually at The Citadel for over a year and a half before I dropped out. Most people think I was there for four days, but I was the only non-cadet to study there for a year and a half."

When I found Shannon, she was upbeat and happy working in education, where she's spent years in teaching and administration. In her spare time she does community theater and improv, where her nickname is "The, like *thee.* When people meet me and hear my name, they say, 'are you THE Shannon Faulkner?' I'm very sarcastic and I have a sense of humor and I will talk to anybody."

She's working on a novel, a fictionalized version of what she went through, and says she's made her peace with everything that happened. "I've had very few people speak out negatively against me," she says. "People are mostly positive these days. I wouldn't be who I am today without it. I would still do everything the exact same way."

In 2018, she returned to the Citadel for the first time since that rainy press conference to honor the late author and Citadel alumnus (and fierce critic) Pat Conroy, who had become a close friend and staunch ally during her legal battle. Shannon showed up that day and for the most part was welcomed as a valued member of Citadel history. Before she left, Sumerlyn Carruthers, then a junior at the academy, approached her.

They hugged, and a tearful Carruthers thanked her, the *The Post and Courier of Charleston* reported. "Without her," Carruthers said of Shannon, "I wouldn't be here today."

August 1995

As Shannon Faulkner was recovering, our existence on the Army base became all about preparing for mid-tests. They were coming up fast, and the trainers never let us forget it.

What we all wanted to know, what we were dying to

hear, was how we were measuring up. *How are we doing? Is this what you expected? Are we amazing? Do we suck? Tell us!* The answer was always the same: *Fine. It's FINE. We'll know when the data is analyzed. Keep going. Go harder. Do better. Get stronger.*

They would expound only about one extraordinary result of their experiment. When I sat with them for interviews, they marveled at our tight friendships. "That wasn't in the plan," Pete, always with a soft-spoken way about him, would say back then, shaking his head. "The bonding was more than we'd ever expected—or ever seen."

We were close, yes, but we had our tense moments. One day as I practiced a deadlift—something I still find hard to do correctly—I heard a blood-curdling scream from across the room, at which point my own ear-splitting scream increased the noise.

"Mother*fucker*," I shouted when I dropped the bar on my toe. "Who was that? Who's yelling?" I was limping to shake off the pain.

"You are," Eric said as he passed me to go check on the other screamer.

I hobbled behind him. We found everybody in one piece. Nadine and Amanda were watching Elle on the bench press. The rest rallied around.

"She did it! The girl went and did it," Nadine was grinning as if her own child had made the honor roll.

Elle's face was contorted with effort, her lip curled over her teeth, as she raised the bar twice more, then set the bar on its rests, sat up, raised her arms, and yelled, "Do what?"

We responded: "Fuck that!"

Eric leaned in and helped her nudge the bar back in its hook.

"One-hundred-forty pounds," Elle laughed as if she'd won the lottery. "*Wow.*"

"More than your body weight," Eric observed. "Not bad."

We all high-fived and hugged Elle. "This calls for a celebration!" Nadine announced. "Who's up for dancing this weekend?"

"I'm up for tequila," I said, "but I don't dance. Under any circumstances."

"I'm in," Elle agreed. "If Eric comes too."

Jean nodded. "Yep. Come out with us." Everett appeared out of nowhere.

"You, too, Ev," Elle said. "Friday night."

The two men shrugged agreeably. "Where?" Everett asked.

"Doo Wops!" I yelled, then turned the music up.

Donna suggested we think bigger. "What about Jillian's?"

We carpooled into Boston, and Elle gamely drove me to Landsdowne Street in her minivan. Everett and Eric arrived separately and blended in with our little group like honorary study volunteers, and we played pool and some of us tossed back tequila shots and all of us joked and danced, even me, because of the shots.

"Next time," Jean winced, "let's do a slippery nipple. Or literally *anything* that doesn't erode my throat like battery acid."

"Marion," I said. "Truth or dare?"

"Truth."

"Why did you join the Army? It seems so dangerous. You could be—"

"Sara!" Elle cried.

"It's OK," Marion said calmly. "*You* can be killed crossing the street tomorrow. I don't worry about that. I just think about my job."

"You compartmentalize," Elle said.

"Exactly," Marion replied. "I guess I joined the Army for the same reason a lot of other people do. My housing is paid for, health care is free, and they'll pay for college. And I get to live and work with people who are willing to die for me."

"We're *all* insane," Jean agreed. "I mean, we signed up for this for five-hundred bucks? What were we *thinking*?"

"I could use five-hundred bucks," Donna replied.

"Your turn, Sara," Elle homed in on me. "Truth or dare."

"Truth."

"Would you ever date our trainer?"

I paused. I took a chug of my beer.

"Come on," Elle said. "You're single, young, pretty… he's single…"

I meant to speak, but spewed a sort of *pffft-shh* sound. The actual answer was, *It's not up to me.* Nadine, ever the intuitive one, ever the caretaker, saved me.

"Billy's cute. You guys make a great couple," she said to Marion.

"He's a good one," Marion replied. "What about you,

Nadine? Anyone new in your life?"

Nadine nodded. "I actually am seeing someone," she told us with a huge smile. "It's going well. I'm happy."

That was all she seemed to want to say right then, so I turned to Donna, who was watching Eric hit the cue ball. "Look—it's our turn," she said before I could ask her anything, and she hopped up to join the guys. That game should have been called Avoid the Question and Don't Dare. We played pool, and then Elle heard a song she loved, and we all danced, and Everett and Eric let loose like I'd never seen. They took turns picking us up and swinging and dipping us and going low, which of course turned into a competition of who had the strongest quads and loosest hamstrings and could dance in a squat for the longest. By the end it was like we'd been out clubbing together for years, and when it was over, I wondered if any other scientists in the history of the world ever went out dancing until the wee hours with their guinea pigs.

10

Don't go, Jason Waterfalls

"That day, for no particular reason, I decided to go for a little run. So I ran to the end of the road.... For no particular reason, I just kept on goin.'" – Forrest Gump

As mid-testing crept up, we were hit with a series of bad omens.

It was a pleasantly warm day when one of the test subjects disappeared. It was no one's fault, though Eric still feels the guilt of it. Change was a part of the study's protocol, and the team kept a sharp eye on morale. When we grew antsy, they flipped the scenery. One day, when it was a tad cooler and perfect weather for outdoor workouts, Eric decided his morning group needed a fun diversion, so he took them to the woods.

"Two miles," Eric told them when they were all assembled in that dusty little lot. "You all remember the route from the trailer pull?"

He stood to the side and hit his stopwatch, ready to follow along, mix in, and monitor their pace. The woods had more hazards than our flat surface on the base, and the terrain wasn't as familiar to the subjects. As in every group, there were the chronically slower runners, the middle-of-the-road girls, and the fast feet. Sienna was a runner. She took off, and Eric kept one eye on her as he jogged past the slower stragglers. They made it halfway through the first loop as a group, and then they hit the meadow. Sienna stretched her legs, felt the wind in her hair, saw the open field ahead and took off. Eric fell back to make sure those in the rear made it out of the woods in one piece.

With the women carrying no equipment nor bearing heavy loads, Eric was fine going it alone in his supervisory role that day. He raced back, found the last few joggers and urged them on. The middle pack moved faster. Eric upped his pace, and the final three women kicked it up a notch. Eric looked up at the front. Sienna, tall and long-legged and easily noticeable, was gone. He sprinted ahead. No sign of her.

The other side of the woods beyond the meadow were silent but for birds and the sound of Eric's own breath. He led the rest of the women back to the start, found no sign of Sienna, and told his charges to stay put. Then he set off at great speed in search of his errant test subject, running, ducking, diving, calling her name. It felt like an hour that he searched, and finally he decided he needed backup and called for reinforcements. There were no cellphones; the team had radios for basic communication. Eric radioed for assistance and got ahold of someone back at the base. Sienna was long gone, Eric explained. She'd missed a turn and kept running, Forrest Gump style, without stopping or looking anywhere but ahead. She ran to make her best time. Sienna was there to fly.

"I can't find her anywhere," Eric said. "She's been gone a while. I'm worried." Our faithful trainer was, in truth, completely panic-stricken, thinking the worst, that she'd been abducted or he was going to stumble on her bloody body. He was, in his words, "scared shitless."

Two helpers turned up to assist in the search, and they fanned out to find Sienna. Finally, at the edge of the park, someone spotted her jogging along the roadside.

"Oh, hey," she said casually. "I got lost."

Eric was nearly overcome with relief. Sienna had lost her bearings and was taking the long way home. It felt like she'd been gone for an eternity, though some estimate it was more like half an hour or so. All was well that ended well, but even a low-risk adventure like that wouldn't fly in this day and age with human test subjects; there are more rules and restrictions now, and they are more stringent. That trip to the woods—and Sienna's detour—would've required Everett to complete a raft of paperwork to justify having been there at all.

Not long after Sienna's mishap, another one of us fell. I tended to stay near the front of the pack on hiking days, and so was ahead of Donna when she went down. It happened fast, with a scream and a *thunk*. She went flying; the weight of the backpack acted as a force to take her down hard. We all stopped, rushed back and rallied around her.

Eric and Ev were by her side lickety split, but our reticent friend, glasses askew and straight brown hair mussed, did not relish the attention.

"Oh God," I exclaimed helpfully.

"This isn't good," Jean agreed.

"Hang in there," Laurie said. "Where does it hurt?"

Two strong arms reached down and pulled Donna carefully to her feet, and Elle and I made sure she was steadied before we let go of her hands.

"She needs to go to the hospital," Eric said to Everett.

"On it," Everett replied, talking calmly into his radio.

"What are you all doing?" Eric whirled on us. "Don't stop!"

Don't stop. The story of our current lives.

"She'll be OK," Ev added. "Two more miles. Stay with Pete and Horace."

"I'm OK!" Donna said with blood dripping down her face.

We moved on, uneasy but determined, because that's what Donna wanted.

I walked into the training room the next day and immediately inquired about my friend. "Ask her yourself," Eric replied.

Donna was sitting on the bench-press bench.

We gathered around our friend, who looked like a raccoon. "You could've taken the day off," I pointed out. "One day wouldn't kill you."

"Why? The hospital sent me home. I'm fine."

She talked a big game but seemed a little shaky. She told us, "I couldn't get my arms up in front of me and I fell on my face. That's where I got the black eyes. I guess I'm lucky nothing cracked open."

Indeed. It was a miracle she didn't lose her front teeth. I hoped that was the last of the bad news, but life never seems to work that way, and there would be more. Not long after Donna was almost catastrophically injured, things went from bad to worse one day when eight of us were full of energy just before mid-point tests. The sky was clear, humidity was low, and the warm air smelled of cut grass. I was innocently lifting weights and sweating too much when Eric called time. That happened often during training—sessions flew by with the quick reps, speed-breaks and chit-chat.

We did a Cement Hill run, and I groaned about it as I always did as part of my ritual, but thanks to Donna I was actually *running* now and was inching closer to a ten-minute mile. There was a bunch of us now who ran together, usually Donna, Amanda, Laurie and I. Nadine would race forward with her impala-like grace, Elle would lope along loosely yet somehow finish near the front, and Marion and Jean were naturals who stayed ahead.

"Not bad," Eric said to me after I came in *maybe* fifth.

"I'd rather get a root canal than run up Cement Hill," I grumbled as I caught my breath.

"We know," he replied. "We all know."

I headed back inside, breathless and thinking about

work. "See you tomorrow," I waved to everyone as I grabbed my things. I had an article due by five.

"That was pretty good today, but we'll give you a killer workout for your last day," Eric called to Donna, using the same tone one might use to comment on someone's new shorts.

"Whoa. Wait. What? Last day? You're *quitting*?" I didn't like the sound of this. "What's going on?"

"I'm not quitting," Donna assured me. "I got a new job. I can't work out at one-thirty anymore."

"Why not?"

"My new job has different hours," she replied. "I was hoping it could work for me to stay with you all, but it's not going to."

"Hey! Congratulations," Elle slapped her on the back.

"Relax. She'll still be here." Eric was puttering about, cleaning up so he could take his break before D-Group stampeded in after work.

"But not with *us*," I hit back. "You'll still see her every day, but who am I going to run with? I can't survive Cement Hill without my running buddy."

"Yes, you can," Eric said flatly. "But I don't think you'll have to."

Jean shook her head next to me. Elle was put an arm around my shoulder and squeezed. "You're faster than you think," Amanda said. "We won't leave you behind."

"I know," I told them. I was grateful for friends who had my back. I turned to Donna. "But I'm not happy about you leaving. At all."

Cement Hill would never be the same without her. C-Group would never be the same. On the way out, after Donna had gone, Laurie said to me, "We'd better do something, don't you think? We can't just let her leave."

"I'm on it," I agreed.

After work, I bought brownie mix, a tub of vanilla frosting and tubes of red and blue icing, and I whipped up a batch of brownies while watching *Melrose Place* from our grand ten-square-foot kitchen decorated in imported beige Formica. When the brownies had cooled, I smeared on an inch of frosting. I opened the tube of red icing and held it over the pan. I thought for a moment, then wrote a brief, special note to Donna in big, jagged, letters. I underlined it in blue. I stood back and regarded my creation. It looked like a fifth-grader's home economics project.

After the next day's workout spent burning approximately 500 calories, I slipped into Eric's cubicle in the back of the room, where I'd hidden 10,000 calories worth of frosted brownies under a sheaf of papers. I jabbed some candles into the dense dessert. Eric poked his head around and whispered, "You ready?"

"Shit. What do we say? Should we sing something?"

Everyone stood around awkwardly as I walked out with the candles lit.

I remember Nadine saving the day. She piped up, "For she's a jolly good fellow, for she's a jolly good fellow…"

We picked it up, all turning and smiling at Donna, who was starting to figure it out as we ended with a roaring, "…which nobody can deny!"

"Okay, girl! Blow them out." I gestured to my weird hand-drawn brownie cake.

She blew them out, then leaned in to see what I'd written. Eric noticed too, and lost his shit. "That's good," he said through laughter. "That's really good."

"*Don't go A*," Donna read aloud. "Ha. I'll try not to."

"Sure, it's funny, but I'm deadly serious," I assured them. Since word had trickled out that A-Group was generating top scores in a bunch of tasks, we'd developed a good-natured rivalry of sorts. "Don't you *dare* go to the dark side."

Laurie asked her, "Have you decided what group you're going to join?"

"I think I'm going to end up joining D-Group. I can go after work."

This couldn't be happening. We hugged Donna through tears and sent her off into her new journey, and Eric stood back shaking his head at our wistful goodbye to a woman who wasn't lost, but was still here, just not in our lives every single day. At the time we didn't know we'd almost lost her entirely. She'd only been in C-Group because her job as a district manager of circulation at the same newspaper I worked for had outrageous hours. "Basically you work in the middle of the night," Donna explained. "If I had open routes, I'd be up at night delivering papers. I'd come home, take a nap and then go to training." But then, "I suddenly had a desk job and it was a much longer commute to Natick. I told them about the study, that I really needed to finish this, and thankfully, they still let me go. I would've been furious if they didn't let me, or if the scientists didn't let me switch groups. There was no *way* I was not finishing."

When we lost Donna, we lost one of our parts. I lost my running partner, and there was one less voice ringing out from our small group in that great room. We soldiered on, of course, and Donna and I were able to remain friends because she didn't join the lovely ladies of A-Group.

Donna was with us on the night of Amanda's 33rd birthday when I found myself stuck in the back seat of a minivan parked on a darkened side street. "This idea seemed a lot more fun during the shopping portion of this excursion. Why are we doing this again?" I squinted.

"Because," a very focused Elle said from the front seat, "It's fun. And Eric will think it's hilarious."

"And we're bored," Amanda added.

There was no denying it. We'd tried to show her a good time, but the pressing sameness of suburbia quickly dampened any hope of real fun. It was the same old thing, just like high school, stuck in the woods and bereft of any cool places to socialize and play or find any action whatsoever. But we all agreed Amanda deserved a killer night out, so someone concocted the brilliant plan of toilet-papering Eric (and Everett's) house in Natick, so we'd raced the fluorescent-light-drenched aisles of CVS grabbing up bargain-brand toilet paper.

"I can't tell if they're home or not," I said. "I don't see anyone in the windows."

"The lights are on, but nobody's home," Donna quipped.

"Let's give it another minute," Marion, who surely knew the ins and outs of effective reconnaissance, suggested. "We don't want them peeking out and catching us."

The radio was crackling in and out, trying desperately to play TLC's "Waterfalls." Amanda started singing along. "*Don't go, Jason Waterfalls…*"

I was horrified. "*What*? No, no, no. You're still young and you need to know these things. It's '*don't go chasing waterfalls.*' There is no guy called *Jason Waterfalls.*"

"OK, OK, it's time," Elle said, whispering now. "I don't think they're home—they could come back any minute. Let's go."

Elle turned off her engine and cut the headlights. We got out, arms loaded with toilet paper rolls, and quietly kicked shut our doors. We spread out and quickly found out there were no actual trees anywhere—so we crouched and fell into a rhythm wrapping toilet tissue around a bunch of bushes.

"I feel kind of bad," Amanda said, weaving more TP through some tiny branches. "I mean, Army women are out there protecting our country and we're in the bushes with toilet paper. I feel like I'm in a bad eighties movie."

"We're well within our rights," I stage-whispered. "After the hell our trainer puts us through? This is the least he deserves." I was rolling fast and sure, like we were being timed and tested.

"No, I mean it's not really fair to Mary," Amanda said.

I paused my rolling. "Mary?"

"You know, that one from A-Group, the one who lives with Eric."

A test subject lives with Eric? Until then, I hadn't heard anything about his new living arrangements. "Wait...the one with the short brown hair? Kind of average?"

"Not average," Amanda replied. "I hear she's wicked fast on the backpack. You should interview her."

Oh, I would. I wrapped faster and harder until my last wisp of paper was spent, then helped the rest of them finish up.

"Eric's gonna *love* this," Elle cackled as we drove off, leaving round, ghostly wraiths in our wake, wisps of paper waving in the breeze. I smiled half-heartedly.

"You OK?" Amanda asked me from the back seat.

"Why wouldn't I be?" I asked.

I was maybe a little jealous, maybe a little angry, and definitely all over the place. Ford was history and Ad Sales Guy was going nowhere since I was too afraid to talk to him, and would in fact veer away from his trajectory if he got within ten feet of me at the office. There were other guys that summer and autumn, including a tall, brooding star reporter from another Massachusetts daily newspaper I met on a night out with the newspaper gang, according to my diary, in which I recorded: *Sept. 12, 1995—He kissed me in front of Kim Girard & a guy named Bob who asked for my #. He took my mind off of Eric, who I only want because he doesn't want me. Fucker.* It was a fun time in a you-never-know-what-could-happen next sort of way, but the boys were a sideshow nonetheless. I'd only been hired full-time at the paper a few months before—I'd been a freelancer for the previous year—and was learning how to cover my own beat while losing half a day to the Army endeavor that was exhausting me physically and mentally. Chasing down stories, performing the maintenance of local news, from cops to town meetings to weather, exercising news judgment, and trying to write compelling copy was a challenge at the best of times.

In the car the night of our prank on Eric, I reached into my handbag, pulled out my new favorite cassette, and shoved the tape in the slot. I turned it up, closed my eyes, and we all screamed along with Alanis's hit song. When it was done, we had a debate about whether we would, indeed, go down on a guy in a theater. I went with no, and one of us admitted she already had. My next favorite was "You Learn." Every line spoke to me. *You bleed, you learn, you scream, you learn.* We are meant to learn from every day, every week, every moment. This time, this experiment, these women. Sometimes the lesson was how basic I still was, how flawed, and how sensitive. How lucky, and how lost.

Eric did not love it, not at all. He did not love toilet paper in his trees, he did not love cleaning toilet paper on his knees. I cannot confirm whether our extra sprints up Cement Hill that Monday were related in any way to our prank, but I had my suspicions. After he showed us our latest workout—we were to lift more now, for far fewer reps, sometimes only five at a time—Eric swept his eyes around the room at each of us.

"By the way," Eric said, "would any of you know about

some toilet paper in my bushes? Because in case you're interested, it takes hours to pick that stuff off. It gets wet and hardens and fucks everything up."

"I do not know anything about any toilet paper," I shrugged.

"Sprints," Eric said.

I set up an interview with Mary for a future article not long after I found out she lived with my trainer. A teacher by day and grad student by night, she was one of our stars. She pulled the trailer like it was fluff and was near the top in the backpack hike. She swears she didn't know she had it in her when she first joined. When she hit the woods for that first backpack test, she was as nervous as the rest of us. She didn't know she had the heart of a lioness and a mind like a steel trap until she faced down Cement Hill and conquered it in a dozen long strides. But she was always tough.

"There's a strong work ethic in my family. You worked hard and you definitely did not complain," she recalled. "We were a blue-collar working-class family. We were mostly happy, although at times we struggled financially. I remember we only had one car growing up and so my mom used to walk me, my two brothers, and sister over two miles each way to the town library to pick out books. It would take much of the day to do this trek but there was never any question or complaints. We just did it."

Those humble beginnings shaped Mary. "I wouldn't have changed any of it," she said. "My mother still has a lot of guilt for the opportunities she could not give us. I look at it so differently. The struggle is part of what made me who I am today. Determination, grit and gratitude are values that have served me well in life."

In our study, with the tasks set for us, Mary could've excelled alone, in the woods or on a mountainside with only the wind whistling around her. But she credits her fellow volunteers for digging down, pulling out the best of her, and surrounding her with beautiful noise. "We got so close," she would say. "They're always there, cheering me on. We were so tight that our friendship became this whole separate thing. I did get in shape, and that was amazing, but there was this big thing happening with this group of women. It was awesome."

As for romance, like many of us, she was half looking, half not, partying a lot, not putting too much stock in brief relationships. Mary wasn't focused on marriage or worried about settling down during the study, but she *was* hoping to have that someday; she craved a roomy, safe house, a "nice home" where she could raise a family and be comfortable, maybe with granite countertops and a yard for the kids.

But for the time being, it was all about the Army and getting strong and supporting her new friends. "Those girls were amazing," Mary would say of A-Group. "We bonded unbelievably. To wake up and those are the first people that you see every day for months? It's *crazy*. To go through the stuff we went though was super hard. I really started depending on the women I was training with."

After losing three pounds in a week and feeling weak from cutting down on proper nourishment, I listened to my trainers and worked to find a happy medium with my food (and adult beverage) intake. I was back to eating when I was hungry, inflicted a certain discipline on night-time grazing, and was rewarded with a continued loss of zero or two pounds per week. I barely paid attention to the scale anymore. What I cared about—as Ev had implored me to do—was how much I was lifting and how fast I was running. I still wanted to drop weight, but not to shrink my body; I wanted to be lighter so I could run faster, last longer, and carry more. This strategy began to pay off, and the day finally came a few weeks before mid-testing when I shut my mouth and ran all the way up Cement Hill for once, then around the bend, ignoring the glances, keeping up with Elle by the lake. I felt free—and then I felt a twinge. Naturally, I ignored it. When I stopped at Eric's timer was when the real pain came, merciless and as hard as a pestle to the mortar in the curve of my hip, grinding, grinding, grinding. I dug my knuckles in to try to work out kinks or relax a spasm or whatever this fresh agony was, and limped inside to grab my things before heading to my car, making sure to stay out of Eric's field of vision. I'd become consumed with the idea of blowing my pre-test times out of the water, and I also knew the team was keeping a hawk eye on their subjects' health.

Injuries in the military—for women and men—are always a consideration when pushing soldiers to their limits. A-Group trainer Chris Palmer, for one, always said it was pointless talk about whether women can keep up physically—because of course we can—but he is nonetheless concerned about the injuries females can sustain with extended extreme physical work. Furthermore, he pointed out that an already strained support system for veterans may not be ready to take care of them if they leave the military with health issues of any kind. "The question isn't *can* women do it," Chris said of opening up all military roles to qualified women, "but are we going to take care of them after we break them?"

In our study, of those who dropped out with injuries, one, a possible stress-fracture on the hip, turned out to be pre-existing. In all, five volunteers left due to injuries related to our training after reporting knee pain, hip pain and sciatica. The hip problem was diagnosed as a possible stress-fracture and the volunteer revealed she had the problem for some time before the study but hadn't divulged it. As Ev wrote in his report, "This greater mean injury risk for females may be considered a reasonable price to pay for the greater talent pool made available by inclusion of women in the military, and fulfilling the goal of equal opportunity for all citizens."

Chris, who holds a PhD in sensory-motor control, has published numerous papers on human performance, and spent years as a programs manager for the Naval Special Warfare Development Group and the United States Special Operations Command (USSOCOM) after the study, isn't so sure. He's seen them go down, watched the strongest men deteriorate under the pounding of a special ops life, watched them limp away after their bodies went as far as they could go. Chris knows how men get injured—and believes, based on current research and his years of experience, that when women start to take their places in the toughest MOSs previously closed to them, they will fall faster and harder. One reason for this is that women are generally shorter and weigh less than men, so the relative load they carry is greater. Further, as Chris explains, "the muscle physiology and anatomy of men and women are different enough" to be a factor in how their bodies react under the strain.

"After years of combat training, we break the men like it's no big deal that they come out of infantry broken—but then we don't take care of them," he says. "So we have men who've been through twenty years of infantry who don't get the service and respect and healthcare they need. Women will be broken down sooner. What are the repercussions? The real move is, no matter what team you're in, that people are used to their best advantage. Let's optimize for the mission and return safely home."

One example of optimizing, he says, is Norway's "Hunter Troop," or the Jegertroppen, touted as the world's first all-woman special forces team. Soldiers in this elite special-ops unit, which would be formed years after our study, train for combat and survival behind enemy lines by cross-country skiing, dragging supplies behind them through blowing snow, carrying packs equaling their body weight for miles, running out of food and going hungry for days, and parachuting out of military airplanes.

"In urban warfare, you have to be able to interact with women as well. Adding female soldiers was an operational need," Captain Ole Vidar Krogsaeter, an officer with Norway's Special Forces Operations, told *Foreign Affairs* in 2016.

Note that the addition of women to its elite ranks is considered a "need" in Norway, not a concession, because that is what our contribution is—necessary. Fifty percent of the population should not be considered an optional pool from which to pull talent to defend our country. "They work extremely systematically and conscientiously, and as a result they often get things done faster than male soldiers," one Norwegian military official told the publication. "If that's related to nature or nurture is hard to tell, but it's the outcome."

A member of the team identified only as "Tora" revealed, "Everyone contributed. When I hit the wall, the others helped, and I did the same for them." Another team member who passed the course in 2016 at age twenty-one told BBC News, "Women think outside the box. Men just do what they are supposed to do. Maybe we are more capable of seeing another solution, a better solution."

The women performed better than men in several key tasks, such as shooting and observational skills. Explains Chris Palmer, "Women's adipose tissue is a higher percentage than men's, so they're more resilient in the cold. They engage in better decision-making in the cold, and you can send out two or three-woman teams and they can do better than men."

Chris has worked with the toughest programs our military has to offer, from infantry to Navy SEALs, and adds, "My personal bias comes in here—equal but different means women don't get less accolades or less pay. We really want to see an equitable society. I've said it for years—you can't count out half the talent pool and expect to win."

I ignored the injury that hit me before mid-testing until I finally *had* to tell Eric, because soon certain movements—squatting and load-bearing were two—made my hip joint feel like it was about to crack like a coconut. He ordered me to scale back on certain tasks. And then, one day, I could barely walk without limping, though oddly I could still run without pain.

"I've talked to Everett," Eric told me. "You need to get that looked at."

I went to take care of it. I visited the doctor and got an X-ray and then an MRI. When the results came back, the scan had found…*nada.* Weirdly, I remember Eric being annoyed when I told him. "Nothing? They found *nothing*?"

No one could tell me why I was in so much pain, and for the first time, I felt like Eric was disappointed in me. That he thought the crippling jabs I reported were not in line with what the experts were saying about the state of my bones and ligaments. What Eric didn't know was that the study had become everything to me. Once I invited it in, it invaded every space around me like wisteria; it had become my social life, my crush, my goal, and my new hope of a healthy body image. Success and results had risen above everything—my old friends, my career, my health. From then on, I did my best to hide my injury. There were still a lot of workouts I could do pain-free. The day after my results came in, we were all reconnoitering at the base of Cement Hill, ready to run.

"Sara. Step aside." Eric waved me away.

I sighed. "Running doesn't hurt," I said. "It never did."

Eric raised his eyebrows, clearly surprised I'd *choose* to run when given a viable out, and that made me realize how much I must have resisted and complained over the past weeks. That day I decided to pretend running was tolerable. That day I finally *found* running tolerable—because it was one of the last training exercises I had left, and I viewed it as a gift. Who would've thought it.

Two days before mid-tests, Eric was torturing us with Cement Hill sprints. "Let's go! *Push* it!" He frowned and held his stopwatch up to the heavens. "Finish hard! Go, go, go!"

I finished ahead of one woman, stopped at the top, bent over, panting, angry.

"Again."

We sprinted up the steep hill again, then walked back down, hands on hips, faces red, lungs stinging. "You can go faster. Go again."

"It's four million degrees out here."

"Line up. I need more from all of you."

Jean was doubled over, panting. "I don't think I *have* any more."

"Then get off the hill. For everyone who's staying: *Again.*"

We all went again, then walked slowly back down, red-faced, dying. Eric readied his timer. "Again."

During a rare break, I asked him, "Shouldn't we be cooling it a bit? Preserving our energy so we don't pull any more muscles? I think I have a full-body sprain."

"You don't have a *full-body sprain*," Eric replied wearily. "This is not the time to let up."

His training philosophy had always been the same. Coaching high school track teams to championship victory solidified his belief that his is the best formula. "The head coaches in high schools are always saying to the girls, 'You got a meet tomorrow—get some rest.' I'm always like, *no*. These kids are never going to get anywhere unless they do the work. There is a time for rest, but *after* you've done a lot of work. My philosophy is that practices are more important than the meets. The meets are just there to see how your practices are going. If you're a shot-putter, you go indoors and get three throws and that's it. At a practice you should get thirty or forty throws, you'll jump on boxes and run sprints, and *that's* how you get better."

He applied the same winning philosophy to our study. "If you didn't do your workouts with the right gusto and frequency, if you were taking the Mayor's Route too often, you weren't going to lift more in the box lift," he told me. "You weren't going to improve. I try not to be an asshole all the time. You can train hard and have fun—but it's not easy."

And so that afternoon, hours before we'd be given one shot to shine, still Eric pushed us. "Again," he said, tensing his fingers around his timer. "This is when it counts. Let's *go.*"

We worked quietly now. Things had gotten deadly serious all of a sudden, and we *got* it, and we gave everything going into mid-tests. They weren't "just" assessments, but an early sign of how final tests would go—the all-important results that would show the Army once and for all what properly trained female soldiers could accomplish.

PART FOUR

LOOK HOW THEY ALL GOT STRONG

11

Desire, despair, desire

I wrapped my hand around the training-room door.

"Hi," said a voice behind me. "You ready for this?" Elle let out a breath.

"Bring it," I said, then noticed she seemed a bit shaky. "Hey—you OK?"

"I have to be, right?"

Mid-testing was happening late due to a mysterious delay we were told had nothing to do with the study, giving us two more weeks of strength training. That extra time brought tensile worry and added pressure to perform even better.

We stormed into the room together. "Hi, Ev," Elle called, loud and confident, and the more I watched her and kept my chin up, and the more I thought I could do this, the more I *knew* I could.

Body assessments were first. I'd instituted a head-in-the-sand policy with the trainers about my waistline, my skinfold test and the DEXA, which was quite relaxing this time—I took a catnap while its lazy arm scanned me. That treadmill test with the name like a Vin Diesel movie was a nail biter for all of us, but we got through it. After so many sprints up Cement Hill and the perpetual suffering of backpack day, the VO2 max wasn't so horrific.

Next, I was asked to jump again, and it was hard to find words to cheer me on with, but my girls gave it their all. It was a *Great try, Sara! Hey, you'll get 'em next time! Look at you…you, uh…made it off the ground! Woo!* I continued to be abysmal at the vertical and the standing long jump. After that, over the following days, I lifted and carried boxes for ten minutes until my lungs burned, and then I did it again without the carrying part as clanging metal and cheers filled the room to the rafters. The pain joined the elation in the air around us, and I inhaled it and used it as fuel. The challenge of squatting in time was *almost* fun now because I was good at them, and keeping time with the red laser helped take my mind off the pain.

When it was time for the progressive standing box lift, we circled up and took turns picking up a box; waiting our turn; adding more weight; trying again. One by one the women dropped out, until three remained at the end—Elle, Marion and I. We hefted the scratched iron amid raucous cheering, whistling and clapping. The din had become necessary, and we'd grown to expect the noise from each other.

We *didn't* expect new voices. As Elle lifted—she was on

track to heft her own bodyweight, a marker of exceptional strength—we heard applause and whooping and whistling through the open door. I turned and saw a group of soldiers and base staff hanging out in the nice weather. They'd congregated by Cement Hill, heard us working, and made their way to our door, where they'd taken one look at us and couldn't help but cheer us on. I elbowed Elle and saw she was already smiling. We received a round of grins and thumbs up from these strangers, and when it was my turn, I wrestled my box onto that pine shelf, using the timbre of their voices to help push it the final inches. They were thawing around here, to be sure. It seemed our determination was finally earning us some respect.

The backpack test was the Big Kahuna, and many of us saw the two-mile trek as a bellwether for our final results. It felt the most *Army* of all the tasks, and it called to that part of us that wanted to conquer every obstacle in our paths. The pack was everything that ever tried to hold us down, and we could buckle under its weight or run with it. It also stressed us out. Some of us heaped undue pressure on ourselves, setting goals to hit times only a highly trained athlete could achieve. I spoke to more than one test subject who felt responsible to perform not only for herself and the rest of us in the study, but for all military women *and* our entire gender.

A-Group's Jane told me, "My biggest fear is, I'm letting everyone down." She *couldn't* let us down, of course; that's not how the study worked. The rat couldn't disappoint the scientist. She is there to be observed, not judged. I knew what Jane meant, though. What is true and what we feel are often two different things.

That morning I made sure to eat what I thought was a healthy breakfast—a small bowl of shredded wheat with skim milk. I ate a banana a couple hours later, and struggled to write a coherent article about controversial water mains in town because every second was occupied by thoughts of the backpack. The load wouldn't press me into the ground this time; it would be light as a feather, because I'd willed it so. I left work early and drove to the woods with a sick feeling and a possibly delusional goal of hitting sub-twenty-four minutes. The backpack had come to symbolize what I *hadn't* accomplished in my life, and it represented everyone who ever told me I was no athlete, who called out cruel names and threw rocks on the playground to try and pop me.

When I stepped out of the Celica, the parking lot was teeming with activity. There were interns and the training team and women from other groups, because tests were scheduled all over the place for those two special weeks. Chris Palmer seemed to be in charge of backpacks. "I'm ready," I informed him. "Let's do this."

Chris barely had a moment to look at me. He was marking something down on his clipboard. "You have a hip injury."

"It's fine. I've been running and everything. Ask Eric."

I did a little walk and a turn for him. "See? Fine."

"You can't even walk without limping," Chris said without a trace of sympathy, but with a clipped, distracted annoyance. "No way you're doing this test. You're out."

I barely knew Chris then. He didn't know me, or my obsession with slaying this test, or how hard I'd worked these four months. He spoke to me like I was…well, an anonymous subject in a scientific experiment. Subjects didn't have *emotions*. They weren't disappointed in mediocre results. They didn't know what mediocre results were. Chris was too busy getting everyone checked in and strapped in their packs to notice my building horror, or to indulge me.

I lasered a world-class evil eye into his back, then stormed off to process at Tantrum Bush, which I'd just dubbed it because that was where I'd gagged and cried so visibly after the last trailer pull. So my hip was killing me with sharp, jabbing, shooting pain and felt as if it were broken. The X-rays and MRI had shown no fracture, so I must be fine. I gathered myself, and thankfully everyone else by those woods was too absorbed with their own issues to notice my quiet rage (and a few stray tears). I hadn't seen this coming, because I hadn't wanted to. The decision had been made well before my encounter with Chris and it was the right one, even if I didn't know it then. I walked out to the head of the path to support my girls. The others lined up, the sound of boots scraping dirt the only sound. It was too quiet.

"Wait!" I yelled. Everyone looked at me.

"Do *what*?" I called.

They answered fast and loud.

"*Fuck that*!"

Eric shouted "Ready, set, go!" and they were off. Everyone started off as expected, with Marion and Elle in the lead. The rest were close behind. I stood on tip-toes, trying to see into the woods, cheering every time I caught a glimpse of a bright-colored backpack. Supporting them was a reminder that life will always go on without you. Sometimes you're the winner, and sometimes you get left behind. If you can take a breath, you are still alive. I waited and bit my nails until Marion finished, red-faced and panting, shaking her head at Chris's offer of help to get her pack off, removing it herself. Elle followed shortly behind, laughing as always: "*Maaan,* that was hard!"

As Horace helped Elle dump her pack, Marion caught her breath.

"They're not far behind," she huffed. "A couple are stuck in Hell Meadow."

Laurie, it seemed, was humping along, not far behind Amanda, and then…*something.* A moment. A butterfly's wing flapped and everything changed. A toe catches a pebble or stubs a lumpy root, gravity does the rest, and the force of 75 pounds takes Laurie down into the dirt. I was not there, but it was relayed to me later that the guys surrounded her, quickly assessing, asking questions. Laurie, sunglasses still in place, shook her head. "Let me up. I want to finish! *Please.*"

The team always did well to balance the need for safety and caution with the subjects' fortitude and heart, and that day was no different.

"You're *sure* you're ok?" One of the team asked.

"It can't end like this," Laurie insisted. "*Please.*"

The men listened to her. Hands reached down, and Laurie took them, pulled herself back on her feet, and kept moving, achy and shaky from a frightening spill. She'd lost precious moments and was now dead last. Like a terrifying game of telephone, word was trickling back to the parking lot, radios crackling and voices raised. *Laurie's gone down! Laurie's gone down? What happened?*

As the last woman hit the finish line, we gathered up, turned back and ran into the forest, some still wearing their packs, to meet Laurie where she was—now at the head of the final stretch. We surrounded her while still giving her space.

"You don't have to do this. I'm OK," Laurie cried.

"No woman left behind," Nadine said.

"OK, Laurie," Elle said. "You lost some time. We're going to run now."

Laurie was sore, discouraged, and exhausted.

"You can *do* this." Nadine's eyes met Laurie's through her dark shades with what was most needed: pure calm. We jogged Laurie in and didn't know that behind her sunglasses, our friend was so touched she was crying. "There was no way I could have considered running that last stretch…but with these friends coming at you, how could I not do it?" Laurie told me a day or so later. She remembers it as "without a doubt one of the sweetest things" anyone had ever done for her. Furthermore, the disappointment of not making the time she wanted was tempered by the fact she still had all her teeth.

The other groups had their own highs and lows. Just because B-Group's Lina was one of the fastest with the backpack didn't mean she didn't suffer. She and the other speed queens, including A-Groupers Mary and Veronica, kept their game faces on in a way I generally didn't. As I wrote in my mid-test article for the *Middlesex News,* Lina was "devastated" to come in second to Mary, who completed two miles in 19 minutes, 44 seconds. Lina finished in 21 minutes and change, still faster than I sometimes ran *without* a pack. She told me about the knots in her stomach before she hit the trail, and I took note of how she banished them. "I'm a machine out there," she said. "I'm just moving the parts. I think of that scene from Rocky II, when he's still in the fight with Apollo. 'I'm not going down. I'm not going down.'"

Mary, who came in first, told me how she shut her mind down to erase the pain, and admitted that finishing an agonizing course had become "a rush" for her. She'd taken the pain and shaped it into something useful.

I was in agony, too, but not from the backpack. I wrote in my diary that day: *I was soooo upset—crying—this week. I'm hurt and can't do the study. Eric and I had a bet going. If I got under 24 minutes on the backpack, he had to get on his knees in front of everyone and call me a beautiful goddess. Fuck. I'm serious about a move to L.A.*

The dreaded trailer test was last. It was my kryptonite, which made me want to conquer it more. It was the one exercise we never got to practice. Once I'd removed that belt back in May, I never saw it again. On the day of my second try, I showed up early and sidled up to Eric. "I'm OK to do this, right?"

"Get ready," he said, fiddling with the trailer's belt.

It had been decided I could manage the two miles without risking my health. Hip-wise, the task wasn't much different than our weightless two-mile runs, which never aggravated my injury. As I prepared to take my turn, I knew nothing of what Jean had suffered earlier in the day. I never suspected a thing.

Our newest C-Group member had proved to be a fun addition, the last person to brag and the first to put her head down and work within a team when required, albeit loudly and with an occasional resplendent spray of swearing. Jean had joined us having already created her own twist on our *Do What? Fuck that!* battle cry. Hers was the equally eloquent *Just fucking do it.* When I asked her if she ever thought of quitting, she replied, "I don't know if I wanted to quit, but I often feel like, 'what the FUCK is this?' Just fucking do it! Telling myself that is how I get through."

The day of the trailer pull, Jean was so focused on getting her sleep and performing perfectly that she left home without a vital item: Her inhaler. Her asthma diagnosis was new, so the life-saving medication wasn't on her mind as she strapped on that belt. One of the guys teetered behind her at a slow pedal on his mountain bike, and as soon as Jean tried to run, she felt it. Her lungs grew heavy, she labored to breathe, and then it hit her: There was no inhaler. She slowed, then tried to charge forward again.

By the time she got to Hell Meadow for the first pass, she was gasping for air.

"I had a hard time breathing and I was like, I know I did worse, and I hated it. It was horrible," Jean told me later. "I remember them telling me to keep going, and I was like, 'I have *no* energy. You're not going to get me to do this any faster. I will walk as slow as I need to.'"

She walked most of the way knowing she was scoring *worse* than she had on the baseline tests back in May. Jean wanted another chance. With inhaler in hand, she could fly through those woods, she was sure of it. "They wouldn't let me do it again," she reports ruefully. "I was hard on myself for that. I hate that I held the scores down. I was always really competitive. I had four older brothers, and I played sports. In college I played softball at Framingham State, and after graduation I found a women's baseball team in Worcester. So at the time, I thought, 'This study is awesome. I want to be part of something big.'"

She laughed thinking back at the modest dreams of our youth. "I probably thought five-hundred bucks was an awesome payout, too."

I knew nothing of her struggles as I strapped on my belt and focused on battling my own trailer-related demons. I set myself an unrealistic goal, to which my trainer shrugged and said unconvincingly, "Go for it," because what else was he going to say? I was counting on pure desire and ambition to put me over the top, but it turned out neither one was up for the job.

The belt dug into my tummy as I took off with Eric on

his bike behind me, the wind in the trees, my boot shuffling in the dirt. From the first step this was no easier than day one. The trailer still weighed the same. It still jerked at me, and I still lacked any running talent whatsoever. I tried going faster, using my new muscles and employing my tuned-up stamina, and it worked—until a hill, at which point I should have learned to control the wagon but lacked the patience to finesse it. Yoda would've kicked me out of Jedi training in a hot second. After that, Hell Meadow, thick with scraggly weeds and long grass, added drag to the wagon. By the time I hit the second lap I suspected I wasn't going to break any records. I wanted to blow my earlier time out of the water. I wanted to blast across the finish line as the trainers and scientists clamped hands over mouths in shock.

I crossed the finish line angry. I paid no attention to the time they called out. The trailer was not the cream-puff I willed it to be; it was baggage I couldn't outrun. The gang knew me now, untied me, and stepped back. They forgave me my emotions. In so many ways I was twenty-four going on four, and I knew it, and I hated myself for it.

"You killed it out there," Elle said as I strode out of the way of people. "Don't worry about it! You did great!"

Laurie, of course, was right there with calming words. "You never give up," she said from afar. "That's what matters."

I managed to absorb a bit of their positivity, comforted that these women had my back, always. They loved me just as I was.

Someone said, "How's Jean?"

"What?" I stopped pacing. "What's wrong with Jean?"

They told me what had happened, how hard she'd fought while her lungs seized up. My friend had risked her life to complete the trailer pull. Asthma is no joke, as Eric, who also has it, assures me. Yet Jean went gave it her best shot and walked away more determined than ever to shine in the final test. That was the key, wasn't it: I had to grow up. No more excuses.

I walked it off for a few more moments. I would be better in the final test. I would set realistic goals, and if I didn't meet them, I wouldn't gag into a bush. "Enough blubbering." I turned and yelled to my friends, "Let's get the post-testing party started. I'm on Jello shots. Who's organizing the keg?"

Elle invited everyone, from interns to A-Group to Everett, to her house for a party to celebrate the end of mid-tests. I went over early, along with Jean, Marion, Billy and a tray of Jello shots. Nadine came in smiling, carrying her little girl on her hip, and we all cooed because she was adorable and already one of ours. We all did a quick hit and then the rest of the gang arrived; I could see them through Elle's kitchen window, coming toward the back deck, carrying food and drinks and ice. Eric, Everett, Mary, a few women I didn't recognize, and some I knew vaguely, were descending.

"A quick toast," Elle said, holding up her red cup of beer. Five of us followed suit. "To C-Group and our honorary male members."

"To C-Group," we said, and we drank, and then the doors blew open and everyone was there, crowding Elle's warm kitchen. I offered my colorful shots around, and most people did at least one. I did two more, and they went down like rubbery clouds of happiness. I offered them up to people throughout the party—on Elle's cedar deck, her living room, the kitchen. I did another shot because they were like candy. Before long, voices grew far away and became like distant echoes.

I passed by some of the A-Group girls on the way out. "Hey," said Veronica. "I liked your last article."

"Thanks," I replied, wobbling a bit.

"You heard anything about mid-tests? Like how we did?" Veronica prodded. "I'm *not* about to fail at this. We're gonna show all the men we can kick their collective asses."

Mary said, "They won't know how we did until they crunch the numbers. The data takes time to analyze."

"I haven't heard anything." I'd asked, too, when I started the pre-write of my story about mid-tests. The guys had told me exactly what Mary said: It takes time.

"I think it's obvious we'd do great in the military," Veronica said. "The backpack's not even that heavy."

Mary gave her a drunken side-eye.

"I could be in the *Army*," Veronica hit back.

"You thought camouflage was *camelflage* until we told you," an A-Grouper laughed.

Veronica held out a hand to me. "Give me one of those, will you?"

I gave her my last two shots and headed outside to the

dark part of the deck. I perched up on the railing with my red cup now full of water, and steadied myself, watching my fellow subjects interact like a silent movie through the glass patio doors. Eric brought his beer over to join me.

"Jello shots got to you?" he asked as he leaned on the railing.

"Yep. I needed some air."

I closed my eyes for a moment and realized Elle's house was spinning.

"Yeah," he agreed. "They go down easy."

Eric took a long sip of beer. A bunch of women came out then to get to the keg across the deck from us, where the deck was lit up faintly.

"What about you?" I asked. "You taking a break from female attention? Gotta love the ratio in there."

"Nah," he shrugged. "I saw you out here and thought I'd come make sure you didn't fall over the railing."

"I didn't know you cared." I drank more water.

"I care," he said. I was glad we were sitting in the dark. "About all of you."

"What if my hip doesn't get better?" I blurted.

"You'll get there," he replied. "Keep doing what you're doing. We have to be smart about your workouts."

Elle rushed out onto the deck before things could get too deep. I watched her look around frantically before spotting us in the corner. "Hey—get in here," she cried. "A-Group is doing feats of strength in the living room!"

"Feats of *what*?" Maybe I was drunk, but this didn't sound like normal party behavior to me.

"They're messing around with Chris, lifting him and

bench pressing him and generally showing off."

I had only a vague idea what Feats of Strength might look like, but I wasn't

going to let A-Group win at it. "Oh, *hell* no." I hopped off the railing and said to Eric, "Are you going to let Chris's group get all the glory? Let's go."

I rushed inside behind Elle and immediately saw what she meant. Test subjects were lying on their backs on the carpet balancing Everett on their upturned feet, his arms outstretched like Superman flying.

"Where's the challenge in *that*?" I looked around. "C-Group, where are you?"

C-Group converged, with Elle, Marion I taking on the guys one by one. We lifted Eric with our arms and then our feet, then we carried Everett, and then Everett lifted two women on his biceps, making his upper arms into swings, and he took Jean on one arm and Elle on the other, and lifted them to shoulder height. That research scientist was one strong motherfucker.

We took Sunday to recover—from testing *and* Jello shots—and then it was back to the grind. We showed up Monday ready to pound out our workouts until final testing, when it would really count. When Eric opened his mouth to yell at us to hurry up, we'd already finished.

"Wow," Eric said, eyes narrowed with suspicion. "This might be a first."

We lined up in front of him, no attitude, no chatter, no complaining.

It took him a second, but he rolled with it. "You won't be doing your run today," he said, looking pointedly at me. "We're doing something new."

"Bring it on," I said.

We did P.A.I.N. runs (*Pace, Acceleration, Interval, Never stop)*, in which the last person in line sprints to the front as the others jog. Then the *next* last person sprints to the front, and so on. This changed things for me. I'd *have* to keep up with the fast ones or risk letting my girls down.

"Just fucking *do* it," Jean said, half to herself.

"Circle up, ladies," Elle said. She cocked her chin. "OK, troops. DO WHAT?"

"FUCK THAT!" Seven voices shouted in unison.

Elle stepped to the start line. "*Now* we're ready."

Eric raised his stopwatch. That was the first of several changes we saw after mid-testing. As the days passed, training grew harder, never easier or more tolerable, and I thought, *where* are the mid-term results? There was no way to know if we were on track to cancel that odious Newt Gingrich and his merry band of misogynists or if we were heading for an embarrassing fall when the final results came in. If we would humiliate the very experts who put their faith in us.

For the entire study, Ev and Pete took a two-pronged approach, serving us both inside the lab and out. Everett kept his subjects motivated on his turf and, like a human tube of superglue, exploited our natural penchant for bonding. It was all part of the experiment—it was essential to keep us nimble, always off balance.

"Regular change in the exercise routine was seen as essential for avoiding physical and psychological stagnation," the authors wrote in the final report in 1997. "The periodized progression of repetitions and weight, as well as the regular substitution of exercises, largely fulfilled the need for change."

After 19 weeks of training, Everett increased our lifting from 21 sets four days a week to 51 sets twice a week. This more than doubled the amount of times we'd be picking up hunks of metal and putting them back down again, a change that quickly discombobulated our sinews and joints and muscles. We blinked and everything shifted, and we became sore and twingey and thrown off, which, as anyone who gets too relaxed in any training regimen knows, is a necessary step. Muscles need to be discombobulated regularly. It's how they get strong.

Perhaps more important than that, the guys aligned our exercises to more closely mirror actual military jobs. "For example, most of the lifts in the latter phase [of the study] employed a grip-width on the barbell which was similar to that of a box of supplies," the team wrote in their report.

These scientists meant business. They created tougher versions of drills we were already doing. Early on, we would stand several feet apart and toss fifteen-pound medicine balls while chatting about our day. Now we would do these so-called "explosive lift" exercises, which required "the ability to lift 'ballistically' using rapid contraction of the knee and hip muscles," as Ev put it, using every muscle and extra coordination to throw that heavy-ass ball as high as we could toward the ceiling. We all aimed for the sky, but I don't remember anyone actually hitting the ceiling.

We helped each other through all of it, and Ev watched us limping and straining and decided to throw us a party. Again, not usual protocol for a deadly serious Army study, but something Ev realized could help keep attrition low, which in the end would help him do better science.

"It was really unusual," Eric once said to me. "I give Everett a lot of credit. He created most of the workouts, and he's the one who made those periodic parties happen. He somehow got money to go get food and put on motivational events." One such event was a picnic on the base for all the volunteers. Everett arranged for it to be catered to facilitate bonding and goodwill as we crept toward the finish, and as Eric said to me, "I'll never forget it—there were eight rotisserie chickens, and someone thought it would be fun to throw one of them around."

Like a female reenactment of the beach volleyball scene in *Top Gun* but with grass instead of sand, birds instead of balls, and shirts instead of skins, "We played volleyball with these chickens," Eric would recall. "No one ate them. We were just out there throwing them around. We had a lot of fun that day playing volleyball down by the lake with the chickens flying over the net."

We got to know the scientists over those months, too. Everett, then a divorced dad of two, would bring his kids to events or to the base. Pete would bring his beloved dog, a friendly fellow we took to right away. Briggs, who Pete called "old brown dog," charmed the test subjects, who soon figured out the pup liked olives and spent that lakeside picnic feeding him under the table "like they were going out of style," Pete would laugh.

It was around that time we learned our mid-term results were nothing short of amazing. I met with the scientists and trainers, who told me we were well on track to proving their workout program could help women perform all the Army's toughest jobs, and then I wrote a feature that ran alongside our staff photographer Ken McGagh's stunning photos. The headline splashed across the front page read, *PRIDE AND PAIN: 40 women in Army strength study pass mid-terms.* Below it was a stunning photo of B-Group's Stacey Meninno, AKA The Mayor, in the midst of lifting a box to the conveyor belt.

The day it hit newsstands, Everett stopped me on my way out of training.

"You are," he said, clearing his throat, "a very good writer."

And then he was gone, and I was smiling. I cared what he thought. I knew how much trust Ev and Pete had put in me to convey their important life's work to the public and everyone they knew, and I intended to make their work and ours sing on those pages. I cared *so much* how my stories were received by the people I'd come to view as heroes, every last one: those who conceived it, the ones who implemented it, the ones who executed it.

That day, for the first time ever, young O'Hara stepped out of his booth at the guard's post when he saw me my red car pulling up to the exit, and if I didn't know better, I'd say he nodded right at me and *almost* smiled.

For much of the study, I was blissfully unaware of any control groups. Our study had a couple, including a coterie of males who'd signed up to see how they'd measure up to us. And they were a special bunch.

The study's report was blunt and clear in its assessment of the men who turned up: "The male comparison volunteers…were only tested and not trained. For the most part, males who volunteered for the study were those who enjoyed testing their physical capabilities and who had the confidence that their performance would be good."

Everett explained to me, "You were going up against strong guys. The average man who volunteered to test himself this way expected to do well, or he wouldn't have put himself out there." In other words, we wouldn't be compared to a guy who didn't lift regularly. *Our* typical guy most likely believed he was God's gift to the gym. "They therefore were in large part individuals somewhat bigger, stronger, and more athletic than average males," the report concluded.

Wonderful. It's just as well I didn't know any of that one day when Eric and Everett beckoned me over to the mousetrap as soon as I walked into the training room. The metal boxes were ominously laid out and the interns stood at attention with earmuffs on.

"Sara. Come on over," Eric commanded.

My jaw clenched up. "This isn't on the schedule," I

blurted, which made little sense, because there was no schedule we were privy to. We did what we were told, when we were told to do it. "What? Did I fuck up that bad at mid-testing? Am I having a do-over or something?"

Everett handed me the ear protectors as Eric said to me, "Ten minutes. You're testing with a male control today."

With? Didn't he mean *against*?

"Uh, OK…so…who is this male—"

And then the male appeared, smiling shyly. "Hey," he said.

"Hey, Billy," I smiled back. So I had to somehow perform better than a six-foot-two nineteen-year-old well-built soldier who'd passed who-knew-how-many Army physical fitness tests. *Got it.*

"I'll try to go easy on you," I joked.

"Don't you dare," Eric said without a hint of lightness.

I had my earmuffs on. I stood over a box. I had no time to freak out further. I squatted, lifted, twisted, threw, rinsed, repeated in an endless rhythm, shutting out everything else, blind and deaf to everything but the boxes. I would've given myself a heart attack if that's what it took to do my best. I felt the work in every muscle. My quads, my back, my obliques, my arms. My pinky toe and my elbows and the base of my thumb and my nostrils. When I finished, I had to walk the length of the room to even out my breathing and cool down. When I strode back, hands on hips, chest still heaving, Billy was getting ready to start. He hadn't trained on this exact drill like I had. He hadn't ever tried it, presumably. But he looked expert at it;

smooth, fit, fast, and strong. He finished and didn't have to dramatically walk it off, head down, like I had. He caught his breath and nodded at me. Eric announced our scores.

"Sara—151. Billy—"

This was going to be bad. So what if it was, I realized. I could only do my best, and I had.

"Billy—145." Eric lowered his clipboard.

I might've said "sorry" to Billy five months ago. I almost did then, but I stopped myself. Billy stepped forward. I was ready for anything except what he did. He extended a hand and I took it. "Wow," he said, shaking his head. "You're *tough*."

That was when I felt my power like wet paint on me, cold and sticky and fresh. I had engaged this strong body and I had soared. Billy and I shook hands, and then we hugged. Marion's boyfriend was an old soul, I thought. There is nothing like a man fully secure within himself. Those two were as calm and sweet a match as any young couple I'd known, and I hoped they made it. I hoped they both stayed safe as they advanced in the Army.

Not all of the male controls were so gracious and relaxed, of course, though to be fair to them, they hadn't trained together and were testing in an unfamiliar environment. Still, Nadine remained unimpressed. "When you watched the male control group, the guys stood there with their arms crossed, thinking who knows what," she would point out. "Like, 'I can beat that fucker,' or 'he's a cheater!' or, 'Watch! I'm going to beat you.' It was never about 'come on, we can all do more!' like it was for us women. *We* were always like, 'One more! You got this.' That energy was what I wanted to be a part of. I was so excited to be there. How lucky I was to not only prove we could do this, but that we could do it in such a cool way."

Jane from A-Group also watched some of the male controls and shook her head. "You know that squat test with the laser showing us the upper and lower limits where you had to hit both on the machine? The trainers had the male controls they had already tested, and the men could do this many, and Veronica was kicking ass. Ev and the guys were standing there like, 'oh my God, you're going to beat the males! *Keep going.*' It was so awesome to watch. That was my impression of them—they were always very supportive and I remember Pete saying that one of the side effects of this was, 'we never anticipated how the women would coalesce around each other and motivate each other.' It's so different from training the guys. They were so competitive and wanting to beat each other, and we wanted to boost each other up."

Later, when I was hanging out with Nadine and the guys and asked them for their reactions to what Jane and Nadine had said about the men, one of them pointed out, "Yeah, but the male controls didn't train in between. They didn't know each other."

"So what?" Nadine said.

"So what," I echoed.

Catherine: 2018

It was back to Quantico for Catherine Afton after graduating from both college and ROTC at once. It was a significant transition, but Catherine was becoming accustomed to leaving friends behind, and soon enough she would be too busy to be sad anyway.

Where OCS was conducted in the heat of half of a Virginia summer, The Basic School (TBS) would be conducted in both hot *and* frigid temperatures over a 24-week span. This would be the final indoc. Here, Marines learn how war is conducted, how to fight, and how to lead an infantry platoon. They learn the culture of the Marine Corps. They learn how to be leaders. Despite its name, TBS isn't basic training; this program is about cultivating the leaders who land there.

Catherine puts it succinctly: "It's basically six months where we go into the woods, and we're supposed to learn how to be a provisional rifle platoon commander."

She and her fellow candidates dug deep to do well there, and success was never something Catherine took for granted. "I would start things at OCS and TBS, and I wouldn't know if I would finish," she says. "I would think, *I don't know if my body is capable of finishing this.* And then when you do it, that feeling is amazing."

There was one hike in particular in which Marines carry their loads to the range for training. That trek can be up to 15 miles long, but isn't meant to be a training exercise—it's a commute. Explains Catherine, "It wasn't considered an official hike, so there was no regulated weight. We would carry whatever we were going to use for the week. My total was ninety-plus pounds including my weapon. We'd go miles, and we were never sure when we're going to stop. I was platoon commander so I had to lead the movement up this crazy hill called Cardiac, where many people fall out.

"Cardiac Hill is not that long, but it's very steep. It's one thing to walk forward and use the momentum of the pack, but you can't use momentum when you're walking up a hill. If I fell out it would be very obvious—I'm leading it. When you're platoon commander you're supposed to be setting the pace. I was very nervous, but I didn't fall out. Some did, and I think if I wasn't leading, I might've fallen out."

So how did you keep going? I asked her. "My mind kind of shuts off for most of it. It's not a choice," she replied. "I have to stay in. There's no other way. I will stay in until my legs physically cannot walk. If I fall over and my legs are no longer working, I fall back. I refuse to believe it's anything but mental."

TBS trained Catherine in everything from navigation to martial arts to leadership to weapons, scouting, crawling through mud and dirt, evading the enemy, and lifesaving in combat. Through it all, she learned what she was not particularly good at: Infantry. "That requires a certain personality and a skill with weapons I don't really have," she admits.

Some of her friends gravitated to ground warfare, though, leaving Catherine with a sense of awe. "I don't like to say anything I went through was that hard," she says. "That's why I hesitate to say OCS or TBS were that tough.

IOC [Infantry Officer Course]—*that's* tough."

Still, TBS for the average person would be a hellscape. Catherine kept her head down and plowed through, even when it was so cold that on one of the courses, "there was a layer of ice on all the water and whoever ran it first had to break it."

She can't forget one of the school's signature events. "There's this thing called the endurance course, and it's the bane of everyone's existence at TBS," she explains. "You have forty-five pounds on your back—you have a tarp in there, two full canteens, a camelback of water, a shovel, all this random stuff on your back. You have your weapon. First you put the weapon in your bag and you do the obstacle course, and then we put everything on and we run about 5.5 miles. You have a time you have to hit. The first two miles are a hilly run through the woods, and then all of the sudden the obstacles come. There are things to climb over, ropes to climb up, and all this stuff. Then I get to the cargo net—this wooden thing with ropes hanging on either side, like a lattice for me to climb up and over."

She began climbing, but the weight on her back was dragging her down. Catherine gave it everything but didn't make it over on the first try. Or the second. "At this point I've fallen twice, but I get up again," she recalls. She kept trying, and in the end, "I just climbed up, I was so determined." When all was said and done, she completed the course with a good time.

That saying about falling down seven times, getting up eight? It works for almost anything.

12

I just want some palm trees

We were in a race to the end now. Thanks to the mysterious delay in mid-testing, the second half of the study was actually the final third. It was speeding by like a bike with shredded brakes down a steep hill, too fast and unstoppable. This journey had worked a deep groove in our lives, and it was unthinkable to have to leave it behind. I didn't allow myself to imagine life without it.

That is, except in the longer term, where I had a vague imagining of where my future lay; I was trying to picture the landscape upon which my *real* life would start, because I knew it wasn't New England. I longed for Western mountain ranges and the Pacific ocean. I was over the cold, dark Atlantic where I'd dipped my baby toes since my parents dragged me here from my birthplace in Salt Lake City. With every article I wrote about the study, I thought simultaneously about how I could never leave my girls, *and* of getting away from here. If I had to cleave myself from them, I'd do it in grand fashion. I'd chase my dreams.

When I told Eric of my plan to go to L.A. in October, he wouldn't look at me. He was frowning at the medicine balls as he laid them out, ready to torture us.

"You knew I was going," I reminded him.

"For the *weekend*. I didn't know you'd be gone for a week. An entire week with final testing coming up? That's…" He was apparently too disgusted to come up with the right adjective.

"I've never missed a workout. One—I've missed *one* workout and that was because I was covering a suspected kidnapping." (It was a false alarm).

I had to go whether he liked it or not. As final testing approached, I faced the end of my time in the study bubble. I'd be leaving Eric and saying goodbye to friendships born of an experience no one else could understand. It was time to focus on my future. I could go anywhere. I could survive on very little, with my car and a credit card, until a journalism job came up. It turned out my friend and colleague Rebecca had a pal who could set me up for a lunch with an editor at a major metropolitan California newspaper. Instead of a drab brick apartment tucked behind some bushes in the suburbs, I wanted to live in Melrose Place. I wanted a pool, palm trees, and an apartment door that led directly outside so that when I opened it, I could speak to an adorable guy who was poking his head out of *his* door.

"It's not that you're missing some training," Eric said.

"It's that you're taking a whole week out so close to final testing."

"I told you—I'll work out every day! I'll do the protocol exactly as you tell me."

"It's not the same. It's never the same."

Elle, ever the adventurer, heard I was going and scrambled her husband's air miles for a quick weekend jaunt with me. All the girls were excited for our sojourn, and C-Groupers including Marion, Amanda and Donna drove us into Boston for a pre-redeye dinner. As we sipped wine and laughed, Marion said, "Uh, guys? Isn't your flight in like twenty minutes?" It was.

We cut it so close we had to sprint to the gate with minutes to spare; we cut it sitcom close, as in that impossible scene in *Friends* where Rachel's flight leaves in thirty minutes but she forgot her passport and magically makes the trip from JFK Airport to the Village and back again in time to make said flight. That was us that day.

"You won't make it," the desk staffer told us as we slammed our (paper) tickets on the counter. "You're too late."

"Shit. Shit, shit, *shit*." I couldn't believe we'd been so careless; we'd had so much fun at dinner that time had slipped away. "When's the next flight?" I asked, defeated.

Elle's face was set to trailer-pull mode. Her eyes were steely, she gritted her teeth, and she pointed at the gate. "I have *two days* to get away and then Macon leaves for his work trip. If I don't make this flight, it's over for me. We're doing this."

She turned and sprinted away, and I followed as best I could, and because it was the olden days, our friends ran with us and saw us all the way to the gate. The frantic flight attendants held the door for us and waved us in. "Hurry! Come on!"

We dashed through the door with seconds to spare. "Sit anywhere!" (Said no flight attendant ever in modern times). That plane was half-empty and it was heaven. We spread out and exhaled, and Elle immediately charmed the flight attendants and then asked to fill out a comment card (before the Internet, paper forms mattered), and they brought us two—along with a bottle of champagne from first class because they were so pleased we appreciated them. They chattered away with us as they popped the cork and poured, and came back every few minutes to refill us, and when we landed they took us to visit with the pilots and pose in the cockpit; the photo is quaintly vintage now, evoking a time of innocence and hope.

I thought it was a given you would become dull and shut down when you got married. I thought it was *all over* once you had a kid. Yet Elle was the coolest friend I had, up for anything that didn't go against her morals and her wedding vows. She came from a traditional family and intended to honor her husband 'til death did they part, which sounded like a life sentence to me, but seemed to make her happy. We had non-stop fun in L.A. even when things got bloody. On the way back from Hermosa Beach on that first day, we stopped to gas up our rental car, and somehow the car door and the gas pump conspired to slam me so hard in the eyebrow it cut me so I was bleeding everywhere. Off we drove using a crinkled paper map to Torrance Memorial's ER to get me some stitches.

That night, two naive young suburban women, I with my long hair covering the stitches, hit the Sunset Strip. I told Elle how I'd read all about the Roxbury in *People* magazine, so we found parking and teetered up on our heels, ready to party with Leonardo DiCaprio and all the nineties cool kids. Elle wore a cute sequined dress and I sported a basic LBD. We were dressed like nuns compared to most others behind the rope. We got near the front of the line and a bouncer beckoned us over. "We're in," I whispered to Elle.

"Private event. It's Magic Johnson's birthday party," the bouncer told us.

"Shit," I said. "Sorry, Elle. Let's try the Viper Room." I switched gears quickly, figuring we could pay tribute to River Phoenix, who had died at the venue two years before.

"You coming in or not?" The bouncer beckoned us beyond the ropes.

Apparently Magic Johnson, whose actual birthday is in August, would be delighted to spend his birthday celebration with us, so we were invited to stay. Elle squealed and danced her way in. I took in the velvet ropes and the star treatment and the beautiful people, and finally, I wasn't at Doo Wops anymore. Elle and I met some famous people even before we hit the main dance floor. Bel and DeVoe—from the bands New Edition and Bel Biv

DeVoe—were hanging out, and we got to chatting about making it big and the work it takes to be successful, and they talked about how they always had so much fight in them and they wanted to make music forever. We took photos with the guys and moved inside, quickly splitting up in the crowd; Elle went to get drinks while I checked out the scene. I recognized one young fellow right away, a guy about my age who was making his way through the sea of people, his head shape and signature scarf making him instantly recognizable.

"Hi," I said to Tupac Shakur.

"Hi," he said back, stopping mid-crowd. "How you doin'?"

"Great," I most likely said. It was meaningless chatter at first, and as he shifted to get closer to me so we could talk more, a gorgeous woman came into view, and he ditched me in a hot second. As he turned to follow her I snapped a prehistoric selfie, which in olden times went like this: Hold up the disposable camera, wait approximately three minutes for the hissing flash to kick in, cross your fingers, and press the plastic button.

I ran into Elle again and yelled out the story of meeting Tupac, which impressed her somewhat, and we drank champagne and danced. After saying happy birthday to a slightly bored-looking Magic Johnson, a guy with a short ponytail and brooding brown eyes stopped me for a chat. He was a BMW mechanic from Germany who lived in L.A. We exchanged numbers, and I raced off to find Elle being followed around by two Toronto Blue Jays. They bought us drinks and we hung out until one of the guys suggested we all leave together. Elle gave me the signal. *Nope*—neither of us were going to go anywhere with these randy baseball players, strapping men who looked to be in their thirties. One got handsy with me; I pulled away.

"We'll meet you out front," I told them. "We have to hit the powder room."

"Do you want to say goodbye to BMW man?" Elle asked as we slipped away.

"He's got my number!" I shouted back.

"Is he cute?"

"Adorable!"

We located our rental and Elle swung the car in an ill-advised U-turn on Sunset, and we sped past two confused-looking Toronto Blue Jays standing outside the Roxbury glancing around pathetically, and I felt bad for a second, but I got over it. Elle went back to Boston the next day, and I went on a hot date with the BMW mechanic who suggested I move to L.A. over a plate of nachos. After our date, my brother asked, "Where'd he take you?"

"Some place with a million pool tables…Billiards Billiards Billiards or something."

"How was it? What did you do?"

"We played darts."

My brother laughed until he cried. The joke of how I only played darts at a pool bar remained in our family ever since. I stayed the full week, worked out in Oakwood's gym, ran between the palm trees around the boardwalk at Hermosa and Manhattan beaches, and worked some new journalism contacts. I told the big-time editor all about the strength study over lunch atop a southern California restaurant rooftop, and he responded, "Uh huh." He glanced at the clips I handed him and never asked to see more. He couldn't wait to get away. Our work on behalf of the Army was meaningless to him, as was I. I wasn't crestfallen because he didn't give me a job or even discuss future freelance work—it's how life goes—but because of how dismissive he was.

"That's quite a feather in your cap," he said vaguely, as if someone other than he might find said feather interesting. I noted he chose a fairytale-like simile, referring to the study as something light and airy and inconsequential; just a feather. *I'm not Robin Hood*, I wanted to snap back. *I'm a young journalist, and look at what I've already done.* But I was a woman, and my best work was all about women, and that bored him.

It was no wonder I wanted to escape the New England suburbs after finding life in L.A. to be exactly as I pictured it. Yet while I was chasing California dreams, I missed a party back in Natick that was so extreme, so unforgettable, that Mary couldn't believe what went on. "We call it the Epic Halloween Party," she told me.

"The party involved cops and boxing. It got so wild the neighbors were furious," Eric rubbed it in. "The cops were called."

"It was such an amazing night," Mary went on. "There was serious study bonding. It was one of those parties we'll never forget. It was a costume party and Everett came up, and my friends from home, Eric had friends in, plus college friends and B-group people who had kids and stuff came. I mean, we're in our apartment, and up comes Everett from his place dressed as a Viking. He used bath mats for shin pads. So he's fifty-two, we're in our twenties, Eric is forty, and we had this eclectic crowd. There were so many different kinds of people."

They never stopped having fun, even when things got extreme. "The neighbors all freaked out about us being so loud," Mary laughs now. "The cops came. That really was the *best party*."

Stacey Coady from D-Group concurred, and showed me photos that proved Mary wasn't exaggerating. The images portray a bacchanal unlike any we'd had up until then; they showed people sucking down tequila from an ice luge, Elle in boxing gloves punching someone, blood (probably fake) dripping down people's faces, hugging, drinking, more fighting. I missed it all.

"Honest to God it was the best party in the history of parties," Eric added with no hyperbole whatsoever.

"Did you hear?" Amanda barreled into the training room with days to go before final tests. "It's *bad*."

"What? Are they giving us more weight on our backpack? Did something happen to Everett? Tell us!" Laurie scooted up to hear the news.

"It's Lina," Elle said.

"Is she OK?" Nadine asked.

"The girl," Amanda told us, "went and got herself knocked up. She's *out*."

"Wait. What does this *mean*?" I was horrified. We'd been taking pregnancy tests sporadically, but I paid little attention as I was always in the clear by default.

"She's out. Done. Kaput. *Finito*," Amanda said.

This was gonna hurt. One of our top backpackers, also a top trailer tester, was toast. It felt like her results could've nudged us over a hump, depending how our results turned out. I could see the headlines: *Army gives 40 women a chance to prove their strength; women fail spectacularly.* I said nothing, and saw my fellow subjects were equally nonplussed, except of course for Elle, who had the annoying habit of looking on the bright side and probably thought it was a good thing to be twenty-seven, married, and pregnant.

"Of course all children are a blessing," I made a huge point of saying as an opener, "but I don't see how this can be a positive thing for us."

It wasn't ideal. Denise LePage, a close pal of Lina's and fellow B-Group member, was fuming. "I was like, 'Thanks Lina! What are you *doin'*? You know you shouldn't have been doin' nothin' during the study," she said, referring to Lina's, ahem, romantic activities. "Couldn't she *wait*?"

We'd be OK, of course, and underneath the panic we were truly happy for our fellow test subject. "One volunteer doesn't define us," Elle smiled at me that day and gave me a light punch on the arm. "Who says we need Lina to do right by final tests? We're C-Group. We can pick up the slack. Bring it on."

"No woman left behind," Laurie said. Just like in the military when a woman gets pregnant, the unit keeps working, and the work continues, and the fight will still be won.

Our last few weeks counted down like a doomsday clock. Eric's hose was packed up and the days were now licked by a chilly November wind. The light had changed, and was now bouncing off the lake in a mellow yellow-orange color instead of a bright white. Thanks to the team forcing me to cut back on certain exercises, my hip was all but healed. There was no more complaining, because Cement Hill wasn't going anywhere and I was sick of my own voice. On one of our last weigh-ins, Eric told me I'd lost a total of more than 15 pounds. On the liquid diet a year before I'd lost 15 pounds in a *month.* No one in the room knew my goals, and I hadn't shared my weight while trying to keep the emphasis off the scale, so I celebrated a small victory alone.

The cold blew in as autumn crept toward winter, and with it came illness and inclement weather and delays that pushed final testing still further out in the 1995 calendar. One day in November, Everett awoke to a blizzard enveloping the state and, in keeping with local schools, called off our training for the day. The guys picked up their old-fashioned telephones with their stretchy, tangled cords and called all the test subjects one by one, leaving voicemails on answering machines and waking some of us with shrill rings rattling phones that didn't have "silent" settings. And as that was tapering off, another round of calls began, this time from test subject to test subject.

Said Mary of that storm, "I didn't have work because I

was a teacher, and we didn't have school. We didn't want to miss a day so a group of us got together on the base anyway just to play in the snow." I wasn't there because I had a full-time job and was expected to get to work, snow or no snow, but many of them came to the base out of habit and a stubborn refusal to miss a session; showing up daily had become as necessary as waking up in the morning. And thus proceeded the snowball fight of the century, amped up with newly formed muscles and fast feet to dive out of the way.

"Chris Palmer was there, Elle was there, Eric was there. It was crazy—we were just running around the base [pelting] each other," Mary told me. "Afterward we went to Mel's Diner and had breakfast together. It's those little blips, those little memories, that make it so special. They stick with you."

The trainers and scientists were less enthused about the unscheduled day off—final testing was happening within days, and there was no time for breaks. As soon as the weather abated, training ramped up again, and the test subjects started to feel the end roaring up to us like a portentous wind warning of the next storm to come. Instead of focusing on the pain of backpack day, there was chatter about what to do with our big payday. Five-hundred spare bucks was nothing to sneeze at.

"There's talk of a cruise," Elle said one day. "Eric? You're in, right?"

"I'd go on a cruise," he nodded.

"Talk by who?" I asked. If there was chatter about a

group vacation, I wanted to be in on the planning. Considering what Elle and I had gotten up to in L.A., it was almost frightening to think what carnage we could wreak on a cruise ship.

"Well? Who else can go?" Elle asked our group. Not everyone could take the time off or spare the money; not everyone wanted to go on a bacchanal at sea. Marion was a hard no, as was Laurie.

"I'm in," Jean said.

"I'm definitely in," I confirmed.

"I know some of the other girls are up for it," Elle confirmed. "The more the merrier." Indeed. I wanted to hear who these merry "others" were, but Eric called time, and we met up for more medicine ball throws.

"Work now," he said. "Cruise later."

"This is going to be epic," I said as I spotted Elle on the bench press. "Me, you and Jean can room together, and if someone else from C-Group comes along it'll be four in our cabin."

"Sure," she said, and kept lifting.

13

Lightning crashes

Eric was in his cubicle when I arrived for our last day of training. He deigned to offer me a distracted "Hey," but didn't look up from his papers.

Jean walked in behind me, and I got a "*Hey*" from her. She leaned on a machine and stretched her quad. Amanda was already there, grabbing her weight card out of the cabinet. She managed a half-smile and a nod. I stared at my own card, a week's worth of notes, numbers, reps and weights scribbled in pencil, and felt numb. It didn't seem real. No amount of reminiscing or squeezing my eyes shut or trying to imprint every wall and machine and person in this room onto my memory could make it so.

Elle arrived last, without a hint of gloom. "Hey, hey, hey," she said, bounding along like an aging prom queen on speed, wearing the same tops we'd all agreed to wear today, our *Do what? Fuck that!* shirts. "Are we ready to work out, or what?"

Eric joined us. "Glad you're all so full of energy. We have plenty to do before final testing." Which would begin something like 48 hours from now. I took a good look at my trainer. I adored him; I was addicted to him, and I was dependent on all my workout angels. They challenged me and lifted me in ways I knew I'd never have again. And *that* was the moment numbness made way for reality. I felt as nauseous as if I'd swallowed bleach. The poison of impending loss ran through me, spreading from my toes to my tummy to my head.

I watched my friends start on their machines without indulging in melancholia, and I too went to work. "Marion?" I asked as she moved between the upright row and the squat machine. "Could you spot me?"

"You got it," she nodded.

I went through all my exercises, and finally landed back at the press one last time with Marion. "I'm *done*," I sat upright easily with my new set of abs and grinned, holding up my hands. Marion slapped me a high-five. "My last bench press!"

"Finished," Elle said moments later, rolling off her machine and holding up her hands. "My last time on the vertical."

Eric was standing in the middle of the room, watching over us as always. I checked the clock on the wall, the one that had run my life along with Eric's stopwatch for nearly seven months, through three intense New England seasons.

"Done," Nadine said. "My last medicine-ball throw."

"I don't want to say goodbye," I said out loud, my voice echoing for one of the last times in the great, silent room.

"You don't have to. It's time for your run," Eric said.

"What? We have only fifteen minutes left. It's over," I argued.

"Yes," Jean squinted in the sunlight as he threw open the door. "It's over."

"No, it's not," Eric said. "Follow me."

He led us outside to the base of my nemesis. There was a nip in the air, though I was still in shorts and a T-shirt. We'd started in the chill of early spring, and we were ending with the cool fall days of November. Eric held up his stopwatch to catch our attention, then brought it back to his palm and held his thumb over the metal button.

"Your last run up Cement Hill," Eric said. "I don't want to hear any complaining."

That did it. I looked up that hill, and then back at Eric. I couldn't complain even if I wanted to. I couldn't get air.

Eric paid me no mind. "Ready, set…GO!"

Off we went, putting one foot in front of the other like every other time. I did my usual, not even trying to keep up with our fastest runners as I trundled up the incline that had tortured me for months. I jogged slowly, my main objective now to *never* stop and walk on this course. No one pulled ahead of me. I picked up the pace, and they picked up theirs.

"No woman left behind," Marion said. "Especially on Cement Hill."

A tsunami of emotion I'd been holding back was now

cresting. I wouldn't cry, and I wouldn't stop. I was stronger now, mentally and physically. I ran up the rest of the slope. At the top of Cement Hill we rounded the corner, and we could see the main thoroughfare up ahead. *Ugh.* Various staff, soldiers and officers were collecting in the area. They tended to pay us no mind most weeks now, but sometimes, on a sunny day, they would stop and watch.

I took a nervous breath. *One foot in front of the other.* This is an important day. Nothing will ruin it. *Be strong.*

"Ignore them," I advised through gritted teeth. "Keep moving."

"Al-*right*," Jean pronounced. "We finally got Sara into running." There was some giggling amid the huffing and puffing.

We fell silent. Now there were more gawkers than ever before, and I fought a building anxiety. They were in uniform, in civvies, in jeans. I ran faster. After we passed them and raced down the small slope, I felt my energy drain knowing I had to pass the crowd again, knowing Cement Hill was in my future twice more, admitting to myself I still loathed it and hadn't conquered it—and at the same time, *oh,* how I'd miss it. As we passed Eric on our way to the third and final lap, he was holding his stopwatch like a talisman. He had an odd look on his face, a sort of twisted expression of determination and…was that *sadness*?

"One more," he shouted as we passed. "Own that hill. Come on!"

"One more! One more, one more, *one more!*" We ran in step in three rows of three as we chanted: "*One. More. One. More. One. More.*"

I shouted as loud as I could when we started up the sharp incline, and at the top I realized how wrong I'd been only a few minutes before: I *had* conquered Cement Hill. I felt lighter. For once, that hike up the slope had been energizing. As we hit our stride on the flat stretch, we saw the soldiers again. We were running faster now. The soldiers were watching up like they used to in our first days when they side-eyed us.

I picked up my pace. "I say we flip them off if we get so much as a guffaw."

"I don't think that's what this is," Jean said. "Look."

We did. And she was right. We got smiles and some nods and waves as they watched us, and then they broke away to go back to their work. As we ran past them, I saw pride in their eyes, admiration, respect. It was visible and genuine. We were almost through when I heard a voice behind me.

"Hooah!" someone shouted. I slowed and looked behind me to see a soldier standing alone in the road. There he was, my conscience for over half a year, smiling broadly at me for the first time ever. O'Hara gave us a deliberate, crisp salute.

"Hooah!" I shouted back. No one else responded. I blinked and O'Hara was gone, and maybe he was never really there at all. He'd guarded the gates, kept me alert and on time and wouldn't let me turn around and leave when my doubts drowned me, and now he was gone because I didn't need him anymore.

We ran together, faster now on the gentle downward

slope, and then along the lake, the autumn leaves strewn in our path, the afternoon sun bouncing off the water's surface. We sprinted up to Eric, then passed him. He didn't bother calling a time. As we caught our breath, a few of us exchanged nervous glances. Goodbyes and endings—they are intolerable at the best of times. Everyone went quiet for a moment, and our Eric didn't seem to know what to say.

Nadine regarded him, then came out with the question we'd all been too afraid, too shy, or too focused to ask him all these months. "Do you think we have a shot? I mean, do you think we can make a difference?"

He crossed his arms, and regarded Cement Hill, and then all of us in front of him. "I think," he said slowly, "that you have done absolutely everything possible. All we ask now is that you show up, focus, and give us your best. The rest of it…" He held up his hands.

"But with all the talk of the future of women in the military," I pushed, "and what they're saying about women and…I mean, what if we *fail?*"

"You can't fail," he replied. "Your job is to keep your heads clear, your bodies healthy, and your focus sharp."

That was no answer. We stared at him; he stared back. And then he gave us one last Eric sigh. "You came here and gave everything I asked of you. I've watched you turn into athletes and I've never been prouder. I've never seen anything quite like you before." He cleared his throat. "I'll see you in two days for testing. Get some rest."

Eric walked back toward the training room. I heard the strain in his voice, and I knew he was going to miss us something fierce even if he liked to pretend otherwise. The rest of us looked around at one another, much like we had on that first day, quiet and unsure. I was ready to cry. Amanda was shaky. Jean was gazing off at the lake as if she couldn't bear to look at us. Elle opened her arms and said, "Bring it in, C-Group."

We converged around her, draping arms over shoulders for a tight huddle.

"I love you girls, you know that?" Elle's muffled voice hit us all softly.

"We know," I replied.

It didn't need to be said that there were two weeks of hard testing ahead, and that it would be a chaotic time, and C-Group would be scattered and busy and likely never be alone together on this base ever again, just us, just the one-thirty girls.

"I'm going to miss you all so much," Amanda said. "What am I going to do in the afternoons now?"

"You'll call *me*," Nadine replied fiercely. "We'll go for a walk. Meet for lunch. That goes for all of you. You need something, you want to talk, you want someone to have lunch with or watch the kids, you call *me*. I'm there. For however long, for whatever you need." I knew Nadine by now, and I knew she meant it, and I found comfort in that.

We were all silent for a moment, and then Elle let go of us and we pulled out of our group hug.

I said, "Do what?" My voice cracked.

Elle raised a fist in the air as we all cried out in the quiet, "FUCK THAT!"

I had one last thing to do before final testing began. I needed to cleanse my mind, reset, and prove something to myself. I wanted to say out loud that I was different now and have it be true. I warmed up the Celica the Saturday morning before tests began and drove to Walden Pond for the first time in seven months. I skipped the headphones, running without music for the full, craggy 1.7 miles without stopping. I didn't visit Thoreau's ghostly ruins or think much about anything. When I made it back to the start, I didn't linger or wander to the shore for a stroll or a last look. I slid back into my car and drove home.

Final testing started Monday. Everyone knew what to do and how to prepare this time, and it started off smooth, an orchestra of machinery and limbs, all of it running with the gravitas the situation called for. The body assessments were uneventful. I watched the scale, though the number wasn't much of a surprise.

When it was time for the VO2 max, we shut up and did it. The treadmill, as it turned out, was the least of our worries. It was the monster who'd never actually lurked under our beds. It was twelve minutes of the easy part.

We were different people doing the final jumps and the standing box lift than we'd been in May. None of it was about where to stand or the uncertainty: *Where do I hold the box, how long do I go for, will this hurt?* It was all about *one more*. We didn't think about surviving it; we focused on crashing through it and obliterating what was in front of us. *One more* pound in the box. *One more* inch on the jump. *One more* box thrown on the conveyor belt. *One more* squat. We cheered and we pushed. There were bursts of levity and cries of agony, but we never stopped.

When I stepped up for the repetitive box lift, everything went away. For those ten minutes I was entirely present; I felt in complete control. My mind was steel, my spirit unbreakable.

Testing was going well....and then it wasn't. For starters, B-Group was missing pregnant Lina something fierce, and it felt like our overall scores would surely take a hit. Then came the snows, and the team put off some key tests due to weather, thus delaying the study's completion still further. With Lina out, A-Group Mary's scores became still more vital. The young teacher was poised to be top backpacker and a tough competitor in the trailer tow—but just when it was time for her test, Mary came down with a mean case of strep throat. It wasn't until after Thanksgiving that she was fit enough to go alone out in those woods, still weakened from illness so she couldn't possibly have been at her peak, yet she went out and pulled that trailer to be a top scorer yet again.

Meanwhile, C-Group had our own setbacks. The first one I learned about second-hand. We were testing at different times and with different groups, and one day I passed Elle on her way out. Her face was gray and tensed up, and she was frowning. *Frowning.* "Gotta run," she said. "Good luck in there." And she was gone. I walked in and asked the room, "What's wrong with Elle?"

I asked again when the subjects had left, and one of the guys told me on the down-low, "I guess she and Macon are having problems. She's pretty freaked out. I'm sure she'll tell you about it." Oh, she would. I'd talk to her when testing was over, after the big party at her place and when the chaos died down. We'd go out for dinner and wine and talk it out.

There was more. Eric found himself more furious than he'd been in the entire seven months during the week of the final trailer tow. One member of my group who was always so determined, so quietly competitive, so ready to score high, had a secret.

"Nadine was doing the pull-cart test and runs by me in the woods," Eric relayed to me. "I'm out there working and she goes, 'I've got news! I'm pregnant!' I'm like, she thought I would be *happy*? I was pissed—it affects the study. I was thinking as an investigator, not a friend. You might remember you had numerous pregnancy tests during this thing. You all signed a paper promising not to get pregnant."

It turned out Nadine's new romance was going very well indeed. We won't talk about how she had continued working out while she knew she was expecting, a big no-no under Everett's human test subject rules. Everyone understood and embraced the good news.

Our friend and former C-Grouper, Donna, took her one shot at glory seriously. As with most of us, the waiting to do the big backpack test was the hardest part. She was at the line with what she called "an intense focus and concentration, waiting, standing there going '*OK, who's next, let's do this, let's get this over with.*'" But suit her up they did, and she was off. "I was just laser focused," she would say. "I was watching the ground to make sure I didn't trip."

Eyes down, forward, then down again, Donna moved as fast as she could over the mixed terrain, but never broke out of a fast shuffle into a full run; she was carrying two-thirds of her own body weight, after all. She was killing it to make the two full miles, and then, "I got near the end and I could hear them telling people their times; I could see the end now."

Lured by the siren call of a "good time," the seductive force that led us all to some form of self-destruction, Donna broke into a run. "I got a spurt of energy," she explains. "I wanted to finish with a good time…and I ruined it. I tried running, and it didn't work, and I turned my ankle."

But so much was different now, and Donna knew from her previous tumble not to let the pack control her entirely. "I turned my body so I fell on the pack, so at least I didn't fall on my face," she told me after. "The guys came running over and they were trying to undo my buckles and I was yelling no, no! Pick me up! Those packs were so heavy; I was flailing. It would've been a struggle to get back up. The guy started trying to take my pack off, and I was kicking and fighting. Don't take that off, just stand me up, I was ten feet from the line. So they backed off, and I finished."

"I was *so close*. It was really just a matter of standing me back up and hobbling the remaining feet. Maybe twenty-five feet." Her new group members, arms outstretched, jumping in the air, called her in, and Donna finished with a respectable time and a feeling she'd left everything on that forest floor. She'd never have a single regret about how she'd conducted herself.

My C-Group friend Jean persevered and planned and prepared to kill it on the trailer pull. "Doing that trailer pull in the mid-tests with asthma was really disheartening, so when I went I was really, really not gonna fail." Inhaler in her pocket, Everett behind her with plenty of water even on the crisp fall day, Jean ran her guts out and pulled the trailer like it was medical supplies on the way to save lives.

"I did a lot better in the final. I remember never making that mistake again like I did in the mid-test and always having my inhaler," Jean told me. "In the end, for the final testing, I was gonna kick ass on this. I'm gonna really try and we're gonna break some records."

When it was my turn to face my own final test, I woke up with the oddest feeling: I was going to miss the torture. I hated to say goodbye to the adrenaline, the nerves, the stakes. I pulled my red-and-pink Celica into the old dusty lot and found the usual serious, tense group of trainers waiting for me. I stepped out of the car and headed to the same start line.

"We're ready for you," Chris said, the rough wooden wagon, even less intimidating now, next to him.

All along I'd thought the backpack test was my white whale, the *thing* I needed to conquer to prove I was as strong as everyone else. But it was actually the trailer pull, and now it was time to show my emotional *and* physical strength. I clipped the padded belt over my waist and pulled the strap to tighten it. It was the same trailer, the same belt, the same woods and the same man on a bicycle behind me. What would be different today? My breath; it was deeper. My attitude, my determination, my refusal to stop. My willingness to feel like a failure and keep running anyway. *I* had to be different today.

"Good?" Eric yelled from his bicycle.

"Good," I confirmed, gyrating my hips to test the belt.

I set off at a trot. I heard the uneven crunch of Eric on his bike behind me. I chose trees as my goals. *Run until that oak or until you throw up. Pain passes. Regret lasts forever.* I hit the downward incline, and the trailer got up on my ankles. I was losing control. It heaved over a rock, and jumped at me like a live, bitter enemy. I thought about what Elle said: *Make it your friend. Don't give in to the negativity.*

Here, my head was as important as my legs. It told me how to maneuver and when, and it kept me focused on the obstacles along the way—unseen sharp curves, roots, rocks. I reached Hell Meadow and frustration turned to rage as I struggled through tangled grass and wilting wildflowers, and I kept running. I ran up the final hill like it was the last thing I would ever do. Once at the top, it was flat all the way home. I saw nothing and heard nothing as I used all my body weight to pull, lean forward, drag that weight.

Up ahead I saw the finish, and I saw our photographer Ken rise up out of a bush with his camera. I burst across the line and managed to halt the trailer just before the main road. I unstrapped myself as Chris rushed up to make sure

I was OK, and to ready the trailer for the next victim. I walked over to the bushes. I didn't need long to gather myself. I turned, hands on hips, and came back to the group. Elle wasn't scheduled to be there at that time to say, *Girl, you did it. You're amazing,* so I said it to myself.

One of my last tests was the backpack. I wasn't going to perform anywhere near the top few women scorers, and I'd accepted it. My goal was to carry it faster than *I* ever had. I was never alone in my doubts and anxiety. Jane from A-Group, the former self-described "slug on a couch," recalls setting her own impractical goals.

"It was like waking up for an exam," she told me. "I was worried I wouldn't be prepared or something would go wrong. I'm always anxious on test day. On the repetitive box lift test, I would be cheering everybody on, but when I went myself, I was always, 'oh my god, how am I going to do?' It was the same with the backpack test. Being in the woods waiting for the gun to go off I'd think, I can't wait for this to be over already. I was worried I'd be so nervous that I'd throw up."

I was the same on my final backpack test. I trekked, and when I grew frustrated, I let the feeling sit with me, and swore loudly a few times, but I never stopped. I was suitably different, from head to toe, than I was in May, and I finished well.

Denise LePage of B-Group got through the big tests with a simple but powerful ethos: "Keep moving and *never* give up," she said in her charming Boston accent. "If you want to succeed, you keep working on it, and you get there.

Never give up. Keep running with that pack, or the buggy behind you, but just keep going. It doesn't mattah. *Keep going*."

We did. And as we blasted through to the bitter end, the weather remained unpredictable, we didn't test much with our usual groups, and the team was busy running a serious experiment. Everything and everyone scattered before the final call. I don't even remember my exact last moments; I know there were no goodbyes, and no closure. On my final day on that base I grabbed my keys, took one last look around at the makeshift training room that would be dismantled after we were gone like a movie set after wrapping, and walked back out to my Celica the same way I'd come in seven months ago: Alone, with an odd feeling in my stomach. It was a most unceremonious finale to a once-in-a-lifetime adventure. It couldn't be allowed to stand, so Elle threw a party to mark the end with a bang.

When the night arrived, I was ready for the party to end all parties, one to relegate that alleged Halloween melee to the back of the record books where it belonged. This one would be a sweet goodbye wrapped in a rager to mark the end to our self-sacrifice of blood, sweat and tears. I slipped on my favorite clogs, wriggled into my Levi 501s and donned a long-sleeved cotton top. My fashion sense was basic, careless and comfortable.

There's a saying about people crying into their beers that's meant to be metaphorical, but I actually did it. After a few drinks in Elle's kitchen with my good friends, I spent the middle portion of the final kegger slumped on the deck, my back against the side of Elle's nice new house, sobbing into my red cup of Michelob, tears breaking the foam as they *drip, drip, dripped.* I'd seen something inside the house, something that hit me like a medicine ball to the gut. I hadn't consciously known, not one bit, likely due to a mixture of denial, cluelessness, and crafty feats of hiding by the couple.

It was a catharsis cry. A drunken cry. A hopeless cry. It was kicked off by what I'd seen, but as tears developed into a full meltdown, it was clear I was weeping for everything: the physical exhaustion, the letdown of goodbye, the accomplishment of losing weight, the failure of not losing enough, and from the uncertainty of how to process the end of something that could never be replicated. I come from a long line of overthinkers. Sometimes the brain needs to empty itself of the mess you make of it. I didn't hear the door open, or hear someone move quietly across the deck, until they were next to me. It had been a long time coming, these wracking, noisy, ugly, snotty sobs.

"You OK?" Laurie asked me. "Oh, of course you're not. Hey, hey…"

Eric was in the living room now, lit up behind the patio doors like a movie screen, lifting Mary up by her waist, while she wrestled to pin him. Their "wrestling" was intimate; little moves and looks that told me this wasn't any ordinary subject/trainer/roommate relationship. My sobs came harder.

"What *is* it?" Laurie asked, extending an arm, letting me lean on her shoulder, and hugging me as I cried. "Let it all out."

She was astute, and she was correct—I was letting it *all* out. *All* seven months of doubt and pain and effort and heartbreak and even victory. I had so much to look forward to, I had opportunity stretching all the way to California, but I was so lost. I felt untethered and bad at being a grownup. I had revved up my career, but it hadn't fixed anything, and no other newspapers would look twice at me. All I could think was, *Now what?* How could I want to leave here so badly while wanting to stay with these people so, so much?

After a minute, I lifted my head slightly to sniffle. "Nothing's turning out like I thought. This isn't how it was supposed to go."

Laurie pulled a tissue out of her pocket. "Isn't it, though?" She asked, pulling back slightly to look me in the eye. "How was it 'supposed' to go? You joined this crazy thing, and you had to know you'd evolve, and change…for the better. It's like going into a cocoon and coming out a beautiful butterfly."

I chuckled, somehow. "I've got news for you, Laurie: You're still the same wise, perfect person you always were."

"*Perfect*? Are you kidding me? I've learned more from this experiment than anyone, I bet," she insisted. "About women, about myself, about *people*. Every day we astounded ourselves. You all put up a prism and shined a light through it to show me what I could do…and then I *did* it. *We* did it."

Nadine had appeared, and was now crouched next to me. "Is it that, in there?" She asked, ever perceptive and unafraid to speak truth, nodding her head to the movie screen where the Eric-and-Mary romcom was playing out.

I blew my nose again and tried to get a grip.

"You're only twenty-four. Where would it go? You have places to go. Things to do," Nadine, pregnant and sober though not yet showing, said.

"I do want to leave New England," I admitted. "But I don't know where to go to start my real life."

Laurie laughed, a little chime of a giggle, not unlike the time she accepted the goldfish from her daughter. "Oh, sweetie," she said. "This *is* your life. Welcome to it."

Beatrice stormed up and listened in.

"Why not me?" I whined.

"You're BEAUTIFUL. Stop it," Beatrice said.

"YOU'RE beautiful," I sniffled back.

"True," Beatrice replied.

She was. I was. Laurie was. Nadine was. Mary was. All of us were beautiful, and so, so fortunate to be here.

Elle came out then. "Hey," she said. "There you are! Everyone's about to do your deadly Jello shots. Then some dancing, yes?" She shimmied, got no reaction, then took a closer look.

"I'm better," I smiled, and clambered up to my feet. "Hey. I looked into those cabins on the ship. It's super cheap if we do four in one room. No window."

"Cool," Elle said vaguely. "Now let's get in there—they're waiting for us!"

Mary was there, and maybe Jane, and Veronica and others, and we did the shots, the last things I needed. A-

Group was hovering around Elle again. Eric was steadying me after two more shots while Veronica grabbed Elle by the fridge. "We booked the tickets," she said to Elle. "You just give them your name when you call and tell them we've already reserved your space in our cabin."

"What?" My Jello shot spit-take was more of an ooze-take. "*What?*" Red dribbled down my chin.

The A-Groupers were oblivious to any unfolding scandal. They were moving on to the next room, probably to lift Chris over their heads and march him around like a trophy.

"You're not rooming with *them*?" I left Eric's side and turned to Elle. "Right?"

I'd gone cold. Yet again, I think I'd known deep down something was off. It hit me then that Elle had said things like "sure" and "cool" when I talked about our cabin on the cruise, but never, *I can't wait to room with you. What are the prices? What deck do we want? Who else will stay in our room?* Stupid me.

"Oh, what? Yeah. Uh." She cocked her head as if someone was calling her, the hostess, from another room. "WHAT? Be right there!"

Elle, Jean and I were the only C-Groupers going on the cruise, and I never imagined a scenario where we wouldn't be in it together. That Elle seemed to have gone out of her way to room with another group—and hadn't just come out and told me the several times I'd brought it up—stung. I wasn't even sure how she knew A-Group so well, given I'd only spoken to them at parties, during some tests, and the occasional newspaper interview. This move felt weird and almost cruelly dismissive of our close friendship. I could only guess why she'd done it, but I had an idea. I felt certain in that moment that Elle had fallen prey to high-school drama. Did she think A-Group was cooler than C-Group? Was she ditching me for the popular girls? The absurdity of hearing it in my own head couldn't dampen the betrayal I felt. I felt like I'd never known her at all. I ran out of the kitchen to the deck in search of an ally.

"Nadine? You're driving home soon, right? Can I hitch a ride?"

She cocked her head. "Are you sure you don't want to stay and work this out? I hate to see such close friends end things like this. It's not healthy."

"I'm sure," I said, breaking out into tears again. "I just want to go home."

"You got it," she said. "I'm gonna go get my kid. I think Ev's teaching her about weight lifting. Then I'll say my goodbyes and we're off. Now dry your eyes and come say goodnight with me." She moved inside, but I didn't follow her. I wasn't in a fit state to see any of them right now.

On the way home I asked Nadine, "Did you know? About him and Mary?"

"No." She shook her head. "They've kept it quiet. I'm not even sure there *is* anything there. Maybe it's just a roommate thing."

I shot her a look in the dark.

"Yeah, OK," she conceded. "But I always thought you two should get together. You're the prettiest one." It didn't matter whether it was true. Once again Nadine said the right thing, the kind thing.

"I can't blame you," she added. "You do seem to have a connection."

Clarity broke its way through my beer-soaked brain that night, and it told me there *was* a connection—an artificial one. Our contact was intimate, and the very nature of such prolonged, intense training creates physical and emotional closeness. What other man had ever known my weight and didn't judge it? What other man could touch my back or check out my knee with two light fingers with complete comfort? He guided me through an intimate, special, close experience, one only forty-six women on the planet have ever gone through. Eric and I shared a sarcastic, merciless, playful sense of humor. All of that was true. It was also true that my friendship with him was not quite as special as I thought at such a young age.

I was right about those two. It was at the mid-testing party weeks before when Mary and Eric had their first kiss, the same party where I chatted alone in the dark with him and confessed my deepest insecurities. Like most couples, they told the story with different spin and emphasis. Her way was more vague, natural, fateful: "I just remember shifting from friends to dating at one of Elle's parties," Mary told me. "That was the first time we kissed."

In Eric's version, Mary made the move. It came about thanks to some alleged gentle advances by a certain test subject, Eric said. "Mary wasn't having any of it. She saw what was going on, shooed the woman aside, sat in my lap, and that was the start of it right there."

The scientists began planning an official closing ceremony for the test subjects who had affected them so. As much as they changed our lives, we also changed theirs. My father allowed us to use his health club after hours for the final *final* party. While that event was being planned, the team got to work crunching data and cleaning up after us, and fifteen or twenty of us stormed Carnival Cruise Line.

Eric and Chris, plus a group of test subjects who chose to spend their $500 windfall this way, cruised to the Bahamas in near-hurricane conditions. We took blackmail-worthy photos involving bananas at Jane's bachelorette party in a cramped, windowless cabin. Eric, Jean and I sipped drinks with the captain. Jean and I roomed together along with a couple of D-Groupers, and one night she and I met two corn-fed Midwestern Bretts at the ship's "nightclub" and drank champagne in their suite with a balcony over the ocean (literally my guy was called Brett). Elle and I easily avoided each other on the fringes, ever polite, never dancing or sitting near each other unless it was in a group. All the photos of us from that trip are in groups, at a distance, and never just the two of us. Not like on the airplane or Hermosa Beach or the training room or outside the Roxbury, or anywhere else we'd been together over those seven-plus months. I have no pictures of just Elle and me. On the cruise, she hung with her other, newer friends. I spent time with Eric and Jean and Rebecca the prison guard, and we all had a blast, but it never felt the same again without the one-and-only C-Group back together in full.

Back on land, there was a formal ceremony on the base on Dec. 7 for the test subjects, in which the U.S. Army presented us with an official certificate thanking us for our service and the way in which we "showed exceptional courage, tenacity, and perseverance by engaging in an extremely physically demanding testing and training program." Then, not long after that, came the *unofficial* closing ceremony at my father's health club. We set up chairs on the aerobics floor and Ev and Pete presented us with their own trophies and certificates. Everyone was there, from interns on up, and many of us brought guests to share in this attempt at closure. The four guys stood at the front and called our names, and one by one, each woman walked up to receive her special, *unofficial* certificate. The guys signed them all thusly: Eric Lammi, Head Hoser; Peter Frykman, Top Tester; Chris Palmer, Master Motivator; and Everett Harman, Main Muscle Manager.

When it was my turn, Eric met my eyes. "In honor of courage in the face of Cement Hill, your totally 'vertical' attitude, and the accomplishment of your own personal best top score in the box lift, we bestow you this certificate to of the High Order of POWER," he said, and one of the guys handed me a certificate on cream parchment paper. Every last one of them hugged every last one of us before we left the stage. (Jean's, hilariously, read, "…in the face of Cement Hill, your totally 'just fucking do it' attitude…").

Back at my seat, I saw that under "High Order of POWER," in small print, they'd written *Pretty Outrageous Women Exercising Rigorously.* The certificate listed my top three best-scored events, which turned out to be (shock!) the trailer pull, repetitive box lift, and squats. I'd gotten stronger in every way. When you work a muscle, it is in the breaking down where victory is born. Each fiber has tiny tears, and from there the whole rebuilds itself until it is stronger than ever. My psyche, too, had tiny tears. I learned from every fall, blister and friendship. The ceremony continued, with top performers receiving special recognition. I remember Rebecca, the prison guard, won the most-improved trophy while Mary took home the top backpack award.

And then it was time to party. We were pinballs bouncing off walls; we were midshipwomen on shore leave. We overran the sprawling club after closing time, doing cannonballs into the pool fully clothed, engaging in more feats of strength, a pickup game of basketball, too much drinking, and more mingling than ever before. A, B, C and D groups were one that night. This was our time to say goodbye; it was our release from all the regimented days and our chance to come to terms with the end. This was, once and for all, goodbye to Ev's historic study that we knew would never be replicated. There would never be a band of sisters quite like us.

Somewhere in the middle of our last, raging goodbye, Elle found me in the women's dressing room. I was sitting on a bench in a damp little black dress (I got splashed by cannonballs), and she was standing over me. She handed me a letter on unlined white paper. I took it and read some of it while she was there. It was mostly of the "Didn't we have the most fun? I'm going to miss the laughter" with a dollop of "I'm sorry you're upset" and hint of a non-apology, and that would be fair considering she, and many who knew our story, might feel she had nothing to apologize for. I looked up at her halfway through.

"Elle…"

"I'm sorry. I wish this could just be over. Can't we go back to the way things were? Let's have some fun."

"You still don't get it. Just go."

She did. After she left, I read the end of the letter and I crumbled at her poignant goodbye. *We had highs of the stars and lows of gas pumps,* she wrote, and as I read the words I thought about how we'd flown the skies together, and how we'd lost hours of our vacation to my bloody cut at the California gas station. *I will always be your friend.*

I'd written her a letter too, but never gave it to her. I wrote it in my diary and left it there. It's six pages long and reveals a sort of pained acceptance about our friendship's collapse over a cruise: *I didn't sign up for it, and pay $500, to party w/ strangers on a boat. You had no intention of changing [your room], and then blamed me for it! I made you feel uncomfortable, etc. When someone who calls me a friend treats me like an acquaintance, that's not a relationship I'm interested in.*

I was already pissed off and hurt before this party started, so I bounced back quickly after reading her letter. I went back to the party, which ended in the wee hours on a disgusting note. Around four-thirty a.m., as cleanup was nearly done and a few straggling party animals remained, our once-favorite intern Horace threw up all over the women's dressing room carpet just as early-bird members started trickling in before the club even opened (my father gave keys to certain favorites). And then Horace yelled for his friends to run away, tearing out of the parking lot as we watched them, open-mouthed. This was the guy who had encouraged us throughout, helped wrap our blisters, cheered us on, adjusted backpacks, run alongside us. Now he was just gone, leaving me to scrape up the remnants of his dinner.

And then the test subjects and our leaders dispersed. Just like that, it was over, floating out of my life on a puff of wind like a dream that had come in the night for only a short while. If it didn't end, it wouldn't be as special. If it hadn't mattered as much as it did, it wouldn't hurt nearly so much. Nadine, who had her own feelings to deal with having to drop out while planning for her second child, put words to the feeling of loss so many of us were experiencing.

"I knew it was hard in the transitioning, in ending one thing and starting another," she said afterward. "It was a letdown when it was over. I think the study affected all of us in huge ways, whether we realized it at the time or not. Looking back, all of us will have something from that study that helped us in our lives. Even when you got really bad blood blisters, and even though you were in pain, you got right back. That's part of what we learned, is that the reward is in the giving. If we gave one-hundred-percent, that was the success. There was always something amazing: the friendships, the support, the fun we had. Those things are all miracles in a way."

Laurie, who now manages the team that welcomes and gives tours to visitors to the Christian Science Plaza in Boston and lives by a lighthouse on a rocky peninsula off the Massachusetts coast, seconds that. "As a little girl I watched the first woman run the Boston marathon, and the night before I'd seen on the news a male doctor explaining that it's impossible for the female body to run 26.2 miles," she told me when we reunited twenty-five years later. "As a girl I wondered, 'how do they *know* that? I don't believe that.' I was proud to be a part of continuing to bust through those limitations on women."

Mary channeled the storm of mixed feelings so many of us were experiencing—pride, excitement, grief and hope all at once—into poetry. She wrote an ode to the study, chronicling it from its raw beginnings with Newt Gingrich bellowing in the background to our blisters along the way and, finally, to its bittersweet end. A few of my favorite stanzas:

We lift weights and we run
And we hike for five miles
Did I mention the backpacks
And our beautiful smiles?

The workouts are hard
And our bodies are sore
We've got blisters, pulled muscles
Bruises and more.

But if you ask "Has it been worth it,
Are we having fun?"
The answer is yes
And we'll be sad when it's done.

As for me, I knew what I was made of when I left that Army base for the last time, and I looked differently upon the words of Henry David Thoreau, who claimed Walden's wood long before I first tread on its soft carpet of pine needles: "I learned this, at least, by my experiment: that if one advances confidently in the direction of his dreams, and endeavors to live the life which he has imagined, he will meet with a success unexpected in common hours."

I conquered Cement Hill and stopped apologizing for the way other people see my body. Elle got her abs, Donna learned what she was capable of, Laurie got her groove back, Mary discovered her inner warrior *and* got her man, Eric found his career, Stacey used her extreme strength to change the world, Marion found a way to manage her melancholy, Nadine got her miracle, and Ev showed them all.

PART FIVE

SEND ME ON MY WAY

14

December & everything after

Over the next few months I got together with the gang for the occasional night out. Elle and I remained distant and I'm not sure which events she attended, if any, or how many she planned without inviting me. Eric had a birthday dinner in December that many of us turned up for, and we got a look at his new mullet for our trouble.

Eric and Mary were officially a couple, but still didn't act coupley. I learned their friendship had begun as soon as he moved into Ev's house. At the time, Eric was following an unofficial, half-hearted rule to *not* get romantically involved with any test subjects, so their Natick home became a sort of *Three's Company* for outdoorsy types.

"He was doing a lot of camping and hiking like he'd always done, and he introduced me to the whole concept," Mary told me. "I had a lot of friends who were up for that stuff, and even to this day I have friends still hiking and camping because of that period of time."

Eric, still logical and blunt above all else, even at the expense of modesty, remembers the beginning of their romance this way: "We started to get to know each other over breakfast. I think Mary had a thing for me before we got together, but I thought there were like ten girls in the study interested in me," he explained. "For some reason I seem to attract a lot of girls. I worked in Yellowstone in my twenties, and one person there was like, 'I'd like to find a girlfriend here, but Eric's got them all.' We worked in restaurants and there were a lot more female waitresses than male waiters and bartenders. I'd end up going out with, like, two guys and fifteen women."

That year he kept finding himself alone with Mary when they crossed paths in the morning, when she would eat toast or oatmeal while Eric scarfed down sausage and eggs.

"It started over breakfast," Mary says. "I would get up early for training, and I would come home and have a little time before work, and he was up getting ready to go to the Labs. We started having really good conversations. It turned out we had a lot in common."

Eric continued living there for a bit, but told me, "After your study I mostly did studies with the altitude group. When it was over, I said um, hey, I wouldn't mind continuing to work here, and they introduced me to the altitude group in Palo Alto. They were all guys that had young kids so they couldn't stay up in the mountains. I stayed in Palo Alto and Colorado Springs all summer and after that I'd come and go from home."

In late 2019, Pete, Ev, Eric, Chris and I got together at Nadine's purple house for our first reunion in twenty-four years. I talked with all the guys about how many military studies had mass bonding like hours. Life-long promises kept like ours. Civilians like ours.

"We had some pretty good bonding on Pike's Peak stuck at the top of a mountain," Eric replied. "At 14,000 feet you can't go anywhere and you're there for thirty days. They had already done sea-level testing in Palo Alto for thirty days. Then they all shipped out to Colorado Springs in Pike's Peak, sleeping together the whole time."

But, I said.

But, he added. "The bonding you guys did was miraculous. I did not expect it."

Everett's team revealed the study's key findings in January of 1996, and what do you know? We blew it out of the water. Our results were blasted out to the national media as a raging success, and a bunch of us did television and print interviews, proudly sharing what we'd gone through.

Key findings included: 78 percent of subjects could now qualify for Army jobs categorized as "very heavy," in which soldiers must occasionally lift 100 pounds, whereas only 24 percent could at the beginning. We showed a 33 percent improvement on the 75-pound backpack test, going from thirty-six minutes to 27.5 minutes for two miles. (For context, soldiers generally move at 3 ½ miles per hour and take a ten-minute rest every hour. Most of us went faster than that). As expected, our bodies changed. Subjects lost an average of more than 6 pounds of body fat and gained 2 pounds of muscle (the full report can be found online; see bibliography).

A spokesman for USARIEM acknowledged we'd shown that women's upper body strength can close in on men's. "This project was designed to provide data to answer, 'Can we fix that [gap in strength] through a training program?'" he told me in 1996. "It appears the answer is yes." We provided proof that women could be trained up for the toughest Army jobs, not with endless time and resources, but before work, on their lunch hours, or after work. The Pentagon's reaction to this was lame: "When the results are available to the leadership, they will take those results and see what they will do with them."

There was another extraordinary outcome from our experiment, one planted and tended by the scientists in the form of keg parties and volleyball games and trips to the woods and even Cement Hill sprints. Because of their focus on motivation, Ev and Pete kept their test subjects until the end. Normal dropout rates for physically demanding USARIEM studies lasting at least a few weeks was about 25% for males and 50% for females at the time, and as Ev wrote, "because this study involved heavy physical exertion…over a six-month period, it was anticipated that attrition could be well over 50%, threatening the integrity of the study."

Surprise! It was not, and it did not. Voluntary attrition was extremely low. For example, one woman left because she had four children and a fifty-minute commute each way, and another dropped out due to "heavy work and family commitments" and was very upset she couldn't continue. Pete, with his decades of experience in this area, still marvels at our staying power. "That is *huge*," he says. "That is something."

For my newspaper's big reveal, the editors chose an image of C-Group's Jean lifting free weights, her expression focused and pained, her knuckles close to the camera lens so the weights are front and center. For those who looked close enough, it was tragically hilarious. "I remember being on the front page of the *Middlesex News*," Jean told me years later. "I have it up on my wall at work. And there's this giant picture of me lifting and holy shit, *you can see the number on the weight*."

I never noticed it before, but when I look now, I can discern the engraved digits: "15." I had tears of laughter rolling down my face as Jean recalled her reaction back then. "People must have been like, 'she's *straining* from this weight?' That's what I thought when I saw it. Why couldn't it have been the twenty-five pound one, or the fifty-pound one? I mean, if you're going to take a picture, tell me and we'll use that! I was lifting was *fifteen pounds*. Thank God it wasn't five though."

Worse still, the gang at work noticed it. "My T-shirt said Toys 'R' Us on it, and you could tell what store it was! It was the talk of the store for awhile," she laughs now.

Even after we'd finished, even with our success clearly spelled out for the simplest minds to grasp, some couldn't help but take jabs at our study. Robert Maginnis, who also happened to be involved in creating Don't Ask, Don't Tell—the Clinton-era policy banning openly gay, lesbian and bisexual people from serving in the military—was back with a newspaper article a year later calling our study "suspect" and "bogus." He proclaimed that 50 percent of the population was useless to our defenses. Under President Bill Clinton, he wrote, "the Army has been radically changed to admit more women, even though there is no compelling reason to do so other than to satisfy the demands of political correctness."

In her 2000 book *The Kinder, Gentler Military*, author Stephanie Gutmann, the other writer allowed on-post (albeit for only a few hours) when our work was done in 1995, wrote that we attracted international media attention *not* because we offered blood, sweat and tears to help the Army make positive changes, but rather, the "TV producers were probably interested because this study had better visual potential than say, the experiment on urine retention. With the strength study you could have that always desirable mix of sex and high mindedness—young women running in shorts in an experiment to destroy the myth...that they are 'the weaker sex.'"

Stephanie, my dear, let me say this to you now, twenty-five years later: No one was chasing me around with a camera trying to capture images of me in my shorts, not one single day, not ever, not before, during or after that study.

"You always hear this," Everett sighed back then. "'Why should you invest time to train women when you can get men off the street?' The answer is, you want intelligent people, aside from being physically able. It's not that much of an investment to train them physically. It's more difficult to train someone for (technical jobs). It's a false argument."

So I asked him then: did we change things? Would our work wake people up and help military women? That remained to be seen. When there was someone in power who truly wanted to change things, Ev told me, this study would be there to back up their argument.

When it was over, I redirected my Army energy to churning out bylines. I kept up my workouts, skipped the scale, and seemed to be losing about one teaspoon of fat a week. There continued to be no boyfriends in the New England area, but I had friends, and they were all I needed then.

One day in the spring of 1996, I got a call from the General Federation of Women's Clubs—I'd become the first-ever winner of the Jane Cunningham Croly Award for Excellence in Journalism Covering Issues of Concern to Women for my articles about the study. I broke into the morning news meeting and told Andrea and all the editors who had supported this effort, and later I would thank my reporter friends who picked up the slack while I was out of the office half the day for seven months.

I didn't have any other job prospects, and I would've loved to stay for another few years if the *Middlesex News* was based anywhere but New England, but when that call came from the GFWC, I knew it was time. I did some more recon out West, this time visiting a friend from college in

Phoenix. One of his pals had a slow, twinkly smile, a dimple, a good job, a pool, a love of sarcasm and Hemingway bookmarked on his nightstand. That was it—next stop, Arizona. Before I left Massachusetts for good, I flew to Nashville to give a speech to the GFWC conference, accepted my award for which I remain extremely honored and grateful, and finished up a feature about the study for *Shape* magazine. As I was in my room on moving day deciding whether to save or ditch my Brad Pitt poster (I ditched it), a *Shape* editor called to ask me to mail in a polaroid of myself in tight-fitting workout clothes, making sure to show my bare legs and arms, so I did.

My sister and I hit the road in June feeling like Thelma and Louise without the bad parts, with nothing waiting for us in Arizona but a cheap summer sublet and a few acquaintances. I launched, fearless, and fell into what came. On the way, in some sort of miracle, we met up with Eric and Ev in Atlanta to watch the Olympic track trials, finding them in their seats without cellphones or even email to guide us. Eric, ever sport-obsessed and unsentimental, watched the games with interest and joy, and no perceptible regret that it wasn't him out there. It was the last time I saw either of them for decades, and the last I spoke to any of the test subjects. I had adulting to do and I found it so difficult I had no room for anything else. But I knew they'd always be there for me and, in turn, I'd have their backs until we were all six feet under, or in my case, sprinkled into the waves.

We arrived in Phoenix to discover our apartment was

unsuitable, so the Hemingway guy, who had a new girlfriend when I arrived, invited us to live on a mattress on his living room floor while I looked for a job. In July, I got another call from the photography department at *Shape* asking for my clothing size (I said 10-12) because I was needed for a photo session the following week. They booked my plane ticket and a rental car, and a few days later I pulled into a canyon somewhere in the L.A. vicinity, found the hair and makeup trailer, and sat still as the experts went to town turning me into a model. They dressed me in drab olive khakis, vintage Army jacket and a snug camo top. I was enjoying everything about working for this glossy national magazine: the glamour, the generous pay, the smart, kind woman who edited my story.

My first and last experience as a model was quick and dirty. The photographer had me walk down a dusty trail, stop, then turn and smile as he clicked away. I traipsed around the dry canyon while he gave orders: *Ooh, yes, good. Now take the jacket off. Hold it over your shoulder. Great job. Turn. Smile. Good.* "We're almost done," he said after a few long minutes as he fiddled with the camera.

A make-up person was standing off to the side, ready to touch up my lips or de-shine my nose. She sighed, "What a surprise. The model's late."

No, I'm not. I'm right here. Hello?

"She was supposed to be here by now. These girls." She rolled her eyes. "They're a nightmare." I was still not one-hundred percent clear on the concept of this "other" model. There was no one to ask; I didn't want to ask.

When the October 1996 issue came out two months later, there was a photo of my lumpy back in a billowing jacket, and my face as I turned my head to look back at the camera, on the title page. Inside, there were multiple glossy pages of a beautiful, skinny model posing as an Army trainee alongside an equally gorgeous fitness model performing some of the lifts and moves we did. Apparently the editors and/or the photo department had taken one look at my size 10-12 frame and choked on their kale. Now: when a writer pens a magazine feature, we don't expect to also model for it. BUT. But, this was a story about improvement, building strength and just plain getting healthy, and that was me. I could only assume they'd considered me, or else why the full-body polaroid? The stylist let me keep the camouflage shirt I wore for the session, and it's tiny. I'm an apple shape who always has ample arms and a buxom chest, and this shirt fit me nicely, and it is *small.* But I was still too fat for them. I could jog miles with a sixth-grade boy on my back, but it didn't matter to *Shape*, because I was the *wrong* shape. It hurt a bit at first, but it was more shocking than anything. I was more disgusted than bruised.

(It was never just that magazine, of course. Even now too many women of different backgrounds, races, abilities and sizes are still fighting for equal representation industry wide. As powerlifter and fitness coach Chrissy King wrote in a 2020 *Shape* article, "While diversity and inclusion have become buzzwords within the fitness and wellness industry, mainstream fitness is still very white and very thin." She added, "Moreover, the industry wasn't acknowledging that fitness and movement aren't about having a particular physique. There was very little discussion about the fact that people could enter fitness spaces for reasons other than shrinking, maintaining, or otherwise manipulating their bodies.")

I shook it off and moved on, and the innate confidence that came with completing the study set off a domino effect of risks and rewards and nightmares. In the same way courage is being terrified and doing it anyway, self-esteem is taking the hit, being knocked down, and then getting back up again. You *will* be knocked down, and over, and sideways—repeatedly. None of us gets out of this unscathed.

After the study, I had eight straight years of never being skinny but healthy and always strong and comfortable and utterly at ease telling anyone who didn't like how I looked to fuck right off. The study showed that exercise is brilliant at strengthening your body, but also your confidence and your voice. Everett handed out questionnaires at the end, and the results that came out months later were fascinating: Fully *85 percent* felt better about her appearance, the key point being how she *felt*. It wasn't that we all necessarily *looked* hugely different—it means we *felt* different about our bodies. The same percentage reported increased self-confidence, a massive win considering the amount of failure and pain we endured. About 59 percent reported a positive change in their feelings about other women, a low number I attribute, unscientifically, to the fact that most of us already had an appreciation for our own gender. No one indicated a worse view of women.

Anyway, none of the newspaper editors I met in Arizona, all of them male, were impressed with my work or my award and I didn't even get any freelance work. My savings were draining, I had nowhere to live beyond August, and worst of all, the Hemingway guy and his friends turned out to be a bunch of asshole misogynists who I'm pretty sure have never set foot outside Arizona state lines to this day, except maybe to go to Vegas. Plus, Phoenix wasn't L.A., even with the palm trees. And so, at summer's end, after experiencing the apocalyptic purple skies, torrential rains and sandstorms of monsoon season, my sister and I turned around and drove back east.

I kept running from there, like Sienna in those woods that day, but for years instead of hours. If this were a movie now would be the montage with quick scenes of a life spent in search of that elusive *something* that would make me whole, or OK, or happy or settled….

…I drive back to D.C., cover Congress for a wire service for a week, get a temp job at *U.S. News & World Report* and then a permanent one in the magazine's New York bureau after meeting the Chief of Correspondents at the coffee machine, get promoted, win another journalism award for the Army series, endure fifty terrible dates and five OK ones, be horrendously traumatized by one man and healed by a village of women, get recruited to work at major global investment management firm, go on vacation to southern Spain, meet a funny British man with cute dimples there, get engaged, move to London, become Vice

President of major global investment firm due to what I'm pretty sure was a clerical error, get married, quit VP job, meet the boss of *People* magazine's European HQ, work for him, start putting on weight again, move to Switzerland, keep working for *People* while hiking up Alps and putting on more weight eating cheese and drinking wine, have two miscarriages, move to L.A. and live across from a giant carwash on Santa Monica Boulevard (!), still work for *People*, interview a thousand celebrities, get sick to death of them, move to Connecticut, get first novel published, publicly quit job at *People*, learn I'm hopelessly infertile, and poof, I'd come full circle back to New England.

I stayed for ten years with the same scenery while my husband worked at his dream job. When he left that company, we were once again in search of new opportunities and thinking about the exciting places we could move to. We are still together after a hundred blazing rows and as many chances to split up; all the painful relationships and traumas and mistakes I made before got me here intact. Without those, I wouldn't know that when things get hard, the grass is still much yellower over the fence, and I have to water my own and stay because I've seen who else is out there and they're not for me.

This should be the end; I should be happy, right? I should've kept up my body positivity and maintained balance. In part because of my fondness for occasional sweet cocktails and dining out, and because of my damaged metabolism and other things that happened as slowly as the saguaro cactus grows, I expanded until I felt unhealthy again. I never stopped exercising, never stopped lifting weights and fitting in long walks and cardio, but as my body reminded me, achieving weight loss (as opposed to health or fitness) is 20 percent activity and 80 percent what you eat. Does that make me a failure? Sometimes it feels that way. But what they don't tell you when they spout the truism *It's the journey, not the destination*, is that there *is* no destination. Would the goalpost be the engagement? The first big job? The wedding? The first house, the first kid? Almost never. After the wedding you look forward to the house. From that house you see your neighbor's bigger, better house. When you get the first job you think, *I can go higher*. When will I be the boss? When you're the boss you want a job at a bigger company. When you make six figures you want seven. When you make a million you want a yacht. When you're a size six you want to be a two.

Some of the most profoundly miserable people I ever met were celebrities. A lot of them seem to have everything and feel nothing. There's one who got famous and rich young, then won Oscars and got to the pinnacle of attention and *things* and adulation and opportunity stretching to the next planet, and he sat in his mansion with a wife he wasn't sure he wanted to marry in the first place and he said, *Now what?* He was still him, but with twelve bathrooms and an infinity pool. He had the same brain and the same feelings and the same body and secretly ugly toenails and receding hairline, same parents, same birthday. He set off on a quest to feel again. He visited strippers, warehouses of alcohol and barrels of drugs, and he threw enough money toward gambling to feed ten villages. He visited monks in the North and cheated on his wife. Nothing changed. From what I hear, he's still working on it, like most of us are. The women have it worse. The most beautiful, skinny and talented among them are told they're never skinny or young enough, and that does lasting damage.

The other thing no one tells you is by the time you get close to the alleged final destination, you'll be old, and that place might not be as satisfying as you dreamed. Oh, they try with their *Youth is wasted on the young,* but that is a title, not the whole book, and it tells us very little. Youth lasts for a long time and then it hits a brick wall. One day something sags, and then something hurts. The day you realize there's more behind you than ahead, your heart is twenty-five but your legs and your lower back and your looks are fifty, or sixty, or eighty. You'll kill for one more chance to look up Cement Hill and be able to *decide* to sprint without aggravating your creaky knees. If you end up rocking on the porch of your dreams by yourself or with whoever you hoped to be with, will you think, I've peaked? This is what I've worked for? You don't. You'll live on the memories of traveling and clubbing on Sunset or teaching English in Japan or fostering a child in your town or cleaning up the beach near you or getting to the top of a peak, however you can get there, whatever your means allow. You're remembering how powerful and beautiful your body was when you criticized it and cursed it.

Everyone and their brother has studied happiness. How

to define it and find it has yet to be agreed upon, and the best attempts at it are still not static or universal. There is the fleeting feeling of joy, as in the opposite of sadness, and then there is the state of being a happy person. My tiny takeaway from what the philosophers and scientists and theologians tell us is that the bumper stickers and posters and your mom were right all along: that elusive *something* is about the journey. There are lists about what it means to have a happy life, and the women of the Natick strength study hit all the highest notes: sinking into a cause greater than ourselves; enduring a good dose of discomfort; tight social ties and spending time with friends; feeling our lives are meaningful; going into the woods and then walking among the trees; setting goals and giving everything to meet them; being generous; and volunteering.

In the final round of interviews for this book, I felt a strong sense of a beginning. We talked very little of where we "ended up," but rather where we are and where we're going. Those "30 under 30" lists aren't everything. Let in the mid-life and later-life success stories. You will be different at fifty than you were at twenty-five, but you will not be finished. You will not be worse. You will have learned and loved and lost, and you will know better what you want to do with the rest of your time here.

Love your body now, however it is. Love yourself *now.*

15

Wake up

The full Natick strength study report was made public in 1997 and soon found a home in the Defense Technical Information Center (DTIC), a repository for information and research for the DOD. Our tears and sweat and life-interrupting dedication were reduced to a series of data points waiting in cyberspace for interested parties to cruise by and pluck out.

Meanwhile, the political landscape remained largely unfriendly toward such ideas. There was some progress for military women under President Bill Clinton, but not so much when George W. Bush entered the Oval Office in 2000. With the onset of the Iraq War in 2003, reports of female fighters in peril displeased many in power and, ostensibly, a portion of the American public, prompting Bush to vow in 2005 that there would be "no women in combat!" on his watch. (Keeping in mind anyone in peril is a terrible thing, the problem continued to be that men on the frontlines were paid and promoted for their bravery while women, as a group, were not.)

But the slow machinery of change never ceases grinding, and that same year the National Institutes of Health acknowledged the powerful impact of studies funded by the 1994 DWHRP, including ours. These 134 experiments "launched an era of research to narrow the knowledge gap on protection and enhancement of health and performance of military women," the NIH's report revealed. "Several important assumptions about female physiology and occupational risks were found to be astoundingly wrong." Further, our experiment and others "allowed reconsideration of standards that were gender appropriate and not simply disconnected adjustments to existing male standards. This surge of research has translated into advances for the welfare of service women and the readiness of the entire force."

As our study wended its way through the system over the years, I heard nothing about it and kept it in a special place tucked away in my memory. It took seeing Ev again in the flesh to get me thinking again about what it was all for. In the summer of 2016 I held a book signing for my middle-grade mystery novel *The Underdogs* in Wellesley, Mass. Surprise guests I hadn't seen in decades showed up, and my heart was full to see my former editor Rus Lodi, who hadn't changed a bit. He sat with my mom in the audience until everyone else was gone and we could chat one-on-one. (Side note: In 2019, Rus's sisters, Major General Maria Barrett and Brigadier General Paula Lodi, became the first sisters in

Army history to attain the general's rank. Rus, ever an ally for women in my experience, praised them in the national media, calling them "a great source of pride and admiration our entire life.")

Before that, when the event was nearly over and the last few kids were handing me their books, I looked up to see Everett standing off to the side. I signed my last one, leapt up, and hugged him. I was still a crier, and my eyes welled up as we talked like were still mid-conversation in that stadium in Atlanta in 1996.

"Did our study change the world? Did it help military women?" I asked him after some pleasantries. He cocked his head and paused in the same way he had when I flipped out at the trailer pulls. "You know, I believe it did," he replied. "I've heard that it did."

He hadn't heard many details so I started asking around and heard some positive rumblings, and in 2018 I launched into full investigation mode. At the most basic level, our study's trajectory can be loosely monitored by the dozens of academic papers, RAND and Marine Corps research papers, books and magazines it was cited and included in. Future scientists, researchers and policymakers picked up our thread and sewed it into the fabric of data on women and the military. New researchers snipped pieces and made them their own, taking our data and weaving it into their own work well into 2017, 2019, and beyond.

And then, finally, the small things, the false starts, the tries, the pushing of the rubber-handled wheelbarrow—it all added up. Someone in power stood up and said, *It's time.*

Leon Panetta was sworn in as Secretary of Defense on July 1, 2011, and landed straight in the thick of implementing the repeal of Don't Ask, Don't Tell. Busy as he was, Panetta thought it was as good a time as any to take on another discriminatory policy.

"When I became Secretary, I saw women operating in the field serving alongside their male counterparts, and I could not understand why we would bar a woman from serving even though she could perform the physical duties we asked of others," he told me in a recent interview. "Women did not have access to a number of positions, and they were not fully equal. I just thought everyone deserves a chance to succeed. We don't guarantee success, but you at least deserve a chance."

Panetta, who was President Bill Clinton's chief of staff during our study, ordered a review of current military jobs by top brass in 2012. "They returned with a list of areas where women were excluded that frankly no longer served any purpose," he says. "So I issued an order in 2012 that opened about 14,000 positions that had previously excluded women."

In April of 2012, Panetta hired Monica Medina as Special Assistant to the Secretary of Defense. Almost as soon as Medina—a lawyer who'd also served under President Clinton—alighted at the Pentagon, she understood what her boss was trying to do. "He was saying, 'this is terrible. Why are women still being discriminated against?' And he gets told the military line: OK, 'we'll start opening jobs one by one.' He hires me and I say, 'this is crazy. Let's open everything.'"

Medina got to work researching every aspect of making such a change, talking to sex discrimination and military experts in and out of the Pentagon, doing her due diligence, and stripping away the arguments one by one. By autumn of 2012, she'd started shoring up support. "There was nothing I heard that should prohibit women in combat," Medina, now an independent consultant, climate activist and founder and publisher of the environmental e-mail newsletter Our Daily Planet, says. "So I walked in and said, 'we're gonna change this.' I went to Sandy Winnefeld [James Alexander "Sandy" Winnefeld Jr., Vice Chairman of the Joint Chiefs of Staff] and explained it. He is a brilliant man and he instantly understood the logic of it. If I could persuade him, a nuclear sub guy and the number two person in the military chain of command, that this was a way forward, I knew we had a chance."

Panetta also credits Chairman of the Joint Chiefs General Martin Dempsey, a crucial conduit between the various branches of the military and the White House. "He really understood the sensitivity with the service chiefs," Panetta says. "He really committed himself to listening to them gathering consensus and developing a plan."

This was progress, but for many who'd been discriminated against for far too long, the 14,000 new job openings were too little, too late. In November 2012, the ACLU filed a lawsuit against the DOD on behalf of four servicewomen and the Service Women's Action Network (SWAN), estimating there were still some 200,000 jobs women were banned from even applying for. "Inexplicably, the military continues to run all-male schools and training courses, including prestigious leadership schools like Ranger School, that women can't even apply to," read an ACLU press release announcing an amended complaint a year later. The group shared the story of Jennifer Hunt, a Purple Heart recipient who fought and was wounded in Afghanistan and Iraq and returned home to still be banned from jobs she was highly qualified for.

By then Medina, an Army veteran who had attended college on an ROTC scholarship and was accustomed to taking on the brass from her days in the Army General Counsel's Office Honors program right out of law school, was already knee-deep in doing just that. Much like the military women she was advocating for, she was up for the fight. She, Panetta and their team, which included DOD Chief of Staff Jeremy Bash, cut through the bullshit like a hot knife through butter.

"The Secretary was with me and the Chairman of the Joint Chiefs and the Chief of Staff of the Army were all with me," Medina says. "The Chairman of the Joint Chiefs is saying, 'we can't say with a straight face women don't do this anymore. We cannot say women are not in harm's way, or that they are not engaged in what is considered a front because the front isn't the front anymore.' But we still had battles to fight to get it done."

Naturally, there were detractors, and not just men and conservatives. Plenty of women, Medina says, were uncomfortable with the idea of females charging into war and working so hard to integrate fully into our military. I found that to be the case in my reporting as well. Many feminists view the military as a toxic, male-dominated and aggressive product of the patriarchy not worth joining. They don't want to focus on being a part of a broken world—they want a whole new world entirely.

Maria Santelli, executive director of the Washington-based Center on Conscience & War, summed up some of the dissent this way: "War is not a feminist position," she told BBC News in 2020. "Feminism is life-affirming. Women and children suffer disproportionately through war around the globe. One's equality shouldn't be based on acquiescence, submission to the military."

My own inner conflict was suppressed during most of the study as I strived to keep my objective journalist hat on. If I was anything, I was anti-military, anti-war, anti-killing. In January of 1991, I'd squeezed into the back seat of an old Datsun between two male friends and rode two hours to D.C. to protest Operation Desert Storm. We marched, we raged, we shouted "no blood for oil" and "support our troops—bring them home!" Kites with hand-drawn peace signs flew overhead and caricatures of President George Bush bobbed in the crowd. We flooded Pennsylvania Avenue and stood outside the White House demanding an end to the conflict.

A year later, when the semester ended, my siblings and father—who we used to joke probably has an FBI file on him from his student activist days—drove from Massachusetts to Virginia to pick me up. On the way back, we stopped by the White House. This time I went inside.

A family friend in Bush's cabinet gave us a private tour on a sunny Sunday, and I padded around the empty Oval office on my best behavior, walked the halls of the West Wing, took in the grand portraits and old furniture, then headed outside to play tennis on the White House court. Before long, the president and First Lady Barbara Bush, both huge tennis fans, strolled down to watch and visit with their Cocker Spaniel, Millie. She stepped on my foot, and her little paws on my shoe have always stuck in my memory. When I got home I wrote in my diary, *Let me tell you, I went to the white house & met George Bush. He, Barbara & the dog were standing by the fence watching dad play. He choked a serve!! We met him and shook his hand. His eyes were extra deep set. He turned to me, shook [my hand], & said, "good to see ya. Good to see all of ya." Consummate politician.*

Such is the gray we live in, and so strong the cognitive dissonance and denial humans can sustain. As my study friend Donna told me as we reminisced years later, "I had mixed emotions about (possibly) being the one that would send women into combat, but I always thought that if we women could do a job we should be able to do it and it shouldn't be someone else's choice. If they're fit and they want to, I always thought [female soldiers] should be able to."

Women desired, *needed*, good jobs in the military, and they weren't afraid to fight. A few years after the study I was asked to contribute to the feminist anthology *Letters of Intent* (edited by Anna Bondoc and Meg Daly) alongside Arie Parks Taylor, a staff sergeant who became the first

Black noncommissioned officer in charge of women's Air Force training. In the course of our correspondence, Arie told me why she didn't fear the possibility of combat.

"My Dear Sara," Arie, a Colorado state congresswoman at the time, wrote, "I never carried that seventy-five-pound pack which you and other courageous women labored with...I did learn that no matter what a woman can endure physically, there will always be those who will simply insist that we do not belong in the military. So the load we must bear is much greater than any pack or physical chore." Her load was especially heavy with sexism *and* racism, and she wrote that "being a Black woman in the military in the '50s was a double hazard." The indignities and damage she endured came from every corner, including from a white female sergeant who called her "a worthless Black nigger." Arie explained to me, "Racism was a divisive factor for those of us who should have been natural allies."

Still, with the world as it was, she did not fear heading to the frontlines. "Sara, you must understand that the lives of Black women have always been endangered. The dangers I faced in the military were no more than those I would have had to confront had I made a commitment to share my life with the wrong man," she wrote. Throughout her life Arie encouraged interested young women to enlist, in part because of what she saw as a modern emergence of a "supporting cast" of activists and progressives inside and out of the military fighting for equality. After a life spent in public service, Arie died in 2003.

As things began to change, most of the resistance to

women in combat came from the usual corners, the places where the concentration of power lay. "While I was doing this, John Kelly, a Marine Corps general who became Trump's chief of staff, was our senior military aide to the Secretary of Defense," Monica Medina, who now serves on SWAN's board, remembers. "Every time he saw me walking down the hall toward the Secretary's office I could tell he was not happy about the decision. But he knew it was Panetta's decision to make and that the Chairman of the Joint Chiefs, Dempsey, agreed."

The momentum was rolling downhill now, and in January 2013 Panetta and Dempsey signed an historic order declaring an end to the ban on women in direct combat roles. "They serve, they're wounded, and they die right next to each other," Panetta said at a news conference at the Pentagon. "The time has come to recognize that reality."

It was an extraordinary moment, but this sweeping change would take time to implement. Every branch of the military was ordered to develop new, gender-neutral performance standards for the jobs that were still closed to women—and at the same time were given the chance to make a case for exceptions to be made for keeping certain positions closed. This order presented a breathtaking breadth of scale and a sea of minute details to sift through. Within each branch, from the Coast Guard to the Marine Corps to the Army, "Every job has a number, and it's categorized, and it's in a type of unit. Different units have different categories," Medina explains. "You might be in an infantry unit, but you might be a clerk. They went through and systematically studied every one."

And as they did, some surprising facts emerged. "They were injuring men at a much higher rate because they didn't know which men could do the jobs either," Medina, who by then was overseeing implementation of gender integration as a member of the Defense Advisory Committee on Women in the Services (DACOWITS), recalls. "Sometimes smaller men were needed for tight space jobs. It wasn't always bigger is better. They learned how many men the military was injuring by not preparing them better for the physical challenges of the job."

As the three-year implementation period neared its end, only one branch continued to argue for women to be excluded from certain positions. "The Air Force had pretty much opened everything anyway, and the Navy was almost all the way there," Medina recalls. "The Navy was concerned about berthing, beds and privacy on-ship in small tight spaces, and that was their big argument for the longest time. By the time I got there, the Secretary of the Navy had pretty much worn them down. There were still some Special Forces and Navy SEALS and things like that, just putting out fires. The Marines were the holdouts."

Marine brass, in fact, tried to use *our* study to show females would *weaken* our country's defenses. In his 2013 paper "Implications of Women in the Infantry: Will This Improve Combat Efficiency?" Marine Corps Major Justin D. Powell wrote that the Natick strength study "determined that although an improvement of 50% was made collectively, they only averaged an increase in 0.9 kilograms of muscle mass. The evidence is clear with this minuscule improvement in muscle mass: when at a biological hormone disadvantage, no natural training can overcome it—and in close combat, the consequences for physical inferiority are severe, often immediate and terminal."

There is no detail given as to what particular task in our study the "50% improvement" is referring to. Furthermore, two new pounds of pure lean muscle ain't bad, and more to the point, ours wasn't a muscle-building study. As Everett explains, "We geared up to improve strength without increasing bulk. Bulk without strength can impair physical performance." In other words, it's like criticizing an experiment on jogging for the fact the subjects couldn't sprint fast enough at the end.

In the fall of 2015, in a last-ditch effort to urge Pentagon leadership to carve out some jobs as exceptions to the Panetta policy, the Marines released results of an experiment they said showed women were detrimental to unit performance in most tactical areas.

"The Marine Corps had done a flawed study intending to prove women couldn't get through infantry training," Medina explains. "They had created these subjective requirements—the teacher could decide how long it had to be and make it as long as it took for women to drop out. Secretary of the Navy Ray Mabus put his foot down and said 'no, this study is flawed and we will not be using it. You will be integrating everything.' He got a huge amount of blowback." (Paralleling Pat Schroeder's comments about military men and their daughters, Medina points out

Mabus has three and Martin Dempsey has two, both of whom served in the Army.)

We all knew women *could*, but there were still people wondering if we *should*. As our trainer Chris Palmer pointed out, other considerations remained, including the particular danger faced by women in wartime. "We already know the enemy won't always follow the Geneva Convention," he says. He referenced Jessica Lynch, who was taken hostage in 2003 after Iraqis ambushed the supply convoy she was traveling in, taking the life of Lynch's close friend Lori Piestewa, twenty-three, the first Native American woman killed in combat in the U.S. military and the first woman to die in the Iraq War. The hit broke Lynch's back in two places and crushed her legs and feet. She was sexually assaulted while in captivity.

At the risk of extreme repetition, let me say it again: Women have always been in danger. It was time they were recognized and paid equally for their sacrifices and bravery. Lynch herself, who struggled with depression in the years following her capture, supported the abolition of the combat exclusion for the same reasons we well-meaning civilians did: "For years women have been fighting for our freedom," she told a West Virginia TV news station. "They've been put in those roles anyway."

As I worked on tracking down the ways in which the Natick strength study might have helped military women, I found we had a direct effect on the Army. Our work in 1995 was, in fact, used as a building block to help develop the historic new gender-neutral standards Panetta had ordered. In 2013, when the military got to work evaluating itself in preparation for allowing women in combat roles, the Army embarked on what was called the Physical Demands Study to set the standards male *and* female soldiers would have to meet in order to perform combat military occupational specialties (MOSs). They were aiming for a quick, cost-effective, gender-neutral way to determine which soldiers were ready to train for the toughest jobs including infantry, field artillery and combat engineering.

The U.S. Army Training and Doctrine Command (TRADOC) called on USARIEM to assist in the three-year study. USARIEM's Military Performance Division chief Edward Zambraski would lead the research teams and Marilyn Sharp, who'd also worked on our 1995 experiment, was selected as principal investigator. Our own Pete Frykman was also assigned to the team.

Sharp is a legend of sorts at USARIEM. She started there in 1981 and retired in 2019, shortly before receiving a lifetime achievement award at the 2020 International Congress on Soldiers' Physical Performance in Quebec City, Canada. When I began tracing the impact of our study, everyone in the know replied, "You need to talk to Marilyn Sharp." She'd been working on experiments with women's physical capabilities—including Army pre-employment screening tests in the early eighties—for years. The Physical Demands Study would tear it all up, burn it down, and rebuild from there. "It's a study I wanted to do my whole life," she told me. "I've done numerous things like it in my career. It was very exciting because we finally got the support we needed."

The official remit was to "come up with predictive physical performance tests to determine whether an individual, regardless of gender, will be able to physically perform the job in that military occupational specialty," and the team spent three years traveling, listening and observing at dozens of Army bases to do it right. "We were a traveling roadshow, all over the place all the time, a huge complement of people and equipment," Sharp recalls. "The support we got from TRADOC was unparalleled. I've never seen anything like it."

Throughout the process, Sharp built on previous research—including her own. She recalls early on when a colleague working on the psychological aspects of the new standards "sent me a technical report and said, 'this looks like something you'd be interested in.' The name on my first study was my maiden name. I had to tell her I wrote the report," Sharp laughs now.

To start whittling down the tasks that would eventually make up the new standards test, the team analyzed thirty-two physically demanding tasks soldiers are required to perform in combat MOSs. They observed hundreds of soldiers in field-training exercises, cataloging exactly how long each one took, who was able to perform to standard, and what equipment the soldier needed to complete the jobs. There was one problem, though: By definition, there weren't enough military women available for this part of the study.

"We used active-duty soldiers, but there were no women

in some of those jobs, so we recruited women from other physically demanding jobs, like truck drivers—women who had to move heavy equipment—and we talked them into participating," Sharp explains.

Through it all, she says, our strength study served as a foundation. It turns out we'd been practicing *The Karate Kid* method of soldiering all along, but instead of martial arts moves, our teachers taught us to lift boxes full of nothing and carry them to nowhere, mimicking the unloading of crucial supplies. Jumping up to touch a measuring stick translated to clearing a trench or leaping over a bush, and Marion or Elle lifting their bodyweight in metal boxes was like loading 90-pound artillery shells.

"We used some of the same soldiering tests you did," Sharp explains. "Over the years we'd used those and modified them. The next step in our PDS study was to take some of the generic tests you did and observe soldiers doing them. We observed casualty drags, rushes, sandbag carries, and many other tasks. Army experts described how the tasks were done and defined the performance standard for success." (That said, she adds, the way active-duty soldiers perform those tasks is usually different from how we did them in a lab setting).

When I asked her how she viewed our study's legacy, she replied, "You showed huge improvements in physical work capacity. Not just strength and aerobic tests but in actual job performance, and that was so exciting—as was the fact that in some of the tests you were coming up at the levels of an untrained man. That was pretty cool."

Our own Pete was there the whole time. He'd watched us for seven months in 1995 and then lived his life, and when the time came, he helped shepherd our study into this brave new world alongside Marilyn Sharp. "Marilyn is a unique link between your study and the PDS," Pete says. "This massive Physical Demands Study was a really different kind of thing, but the two are inextricably linked."

Unsurprisingly, in conducting the PDS, Sharp's team found no job or task that could *not* be done by at least one woman. "Everybody should be able to do [certain things, like] ruck march and carry sandbags," Sharp explains. "Then it was a question of, can they do it to standard? Loading field artillery ammunition, where you're lifting these ninety-pound shells and putting them into a honeycomb rack, is a heavy and very difficult task. We had to train people to just attempt to do it. There were many men who couldn't do it, and just a few women who could. There were some women that performed *way* above the average man. There's always exceptional people for a job like that, and that's who you want to identify."

What emerged from all that research is what's now known as the Occupational Physical Assessment Test (OPAT), a battery of physical performance tests that helps the Army match the right soldiers to the right jobs. The OPAT is four tests that can be completed by about 100 soldiers in two hours. The Army offers second chances for the test and has provided a smartphone app to help those who were not able to qualify for their job to train themselves up and try again.

Sharp considers the OPAT project one of the highlights of her career. "There were so many times they were going to [open all the jobs to women] and they didn't," she says now. "You never quite believe it until it happens. I just look at what was happening in society. Women were firefighters and police officers. Women were in just about everything. They can go to the moon, but they can't be in a certain job in the Army? That just doesn't make sense."

In 2017, the Army awarded Sharp the Commander's Award for Civilian Service, and two others on her team, research physiologists and associate investigators Dr. Jan Redmond and Dr. Stephen Foulis, received the Achievement Medal for Civilian Service.

Exactly twenty years after we humped our last backpack on the base, everything changed for military women. In December of 2015, then-Defense Secretary Ash Carter made the final call: The ban on women in combat would be lifted in January 2016—without any exceptions. "They'll be allowed to drive tanks, fire mortars, and lead infantry soldiers into combat. They'll be able to serve as Army Rangers and Green Berets, Navy SEALS, Marine Corps infantry, Air Force parajumpers and everything else that was previously open only to men," Carter said at the time.

President Barack Obama called the move a "historic step forward," saying it would "make our military even stronger."

Retired Capt. Linda Bray, the first woman to lead a platoon into combat all the way back in 1989, was asked for her thoughts. I imagine it as an eye-rolling moment for a woman who'd fought for her country so long ago. "I'm so thrilled, excited. I think it's absolutely wonderful that our nation's military is taking steps to help women break the glass ceiling," Bray told the AP in 2013. "It's nothing new in the military for a woman to be right beside a man in operations."

Pat Schroeder was relieved, exhausted, and validated. "I felt like the young lionesses had finally won their way," she says. "They had really done it. It's just sad it had been so long and so hard and so uphill. Finally it did happen. Finally we made it."

Women have, unsurprisingly, exceeded expectations. As the first women filter through the system, graduate from Ranger school and lead platoons in Marine infantry, Panetta, who now serves as chairman of The Panetta Institute for Public Policy he co-founded with his wife Sylvia in 1997, says, "I haven't had anybody complain to me that women have not worked out. On the contrary. I usually get people who come up to me and say, thank you for making that decision. Not just women, but men as well say, 'I've been in the service and fought alongside women and believe that in every sense they are true warriors on behalf of our country.'"

The fight for equality isn't over, but there are always people who keep pushing, and the battle continues apace. SWAN and the ACLU are relentless. They filed another suit in 2017 targeting, in part, the "Leaders First" policy of the Army and Marine Corps that requires enlisted women to wait to enter combat battalions until two or more "women leaders" are assigned to those units.

In June 2016, the DOD announced transgender troops would be able to serve openly, but as of 2021 they're banned from military service again, a move former Secretary of the Navy Mabus called "the dumbest government policy you could possibly pursue." GLAAD and the National Center for Lesbian Rights (NCLR) filed a lawsuit in federal court challenging then-President Trump's ban; there is every chance that will flip again under President Joe Biden.

And in 2020, advocates for military women were questioning the fairness of the new Army Combat Fitness test (ACFT), which at this writing has already been modified once to become the ACFT 2.0. It is comprised of six events, and figures show failure rates of 54 percent for female soldiers and 7 percent for males during the second quarter of 2020. The leg tucks are harder for many women, and so, in one modification, the 2.0 version is set to allow a plank instead. If fully implemented the ACFT could affect career prospects for many servicewomen. Monica Medina is not a fan, as she wrote plainly in a Tweet in September 2020: "This test should be halted. The Army must show why EVERY person must pass this test to show they are in shape." Women are strong and we can endure, but once again, placing such importance on physical performance to determine career success discounts service members who bring other extremely valuable attributes to our armed forces. In October 2020, members of Congress asked the Army to "pause implementation" of the ACFT pending further investigation.

Like on Cement Hill or Cardiac Hill, like with the trailer pull, no matter how long it goes on and even if you're vomiting or scared or exhausted, there is no letting up. Those lawsuits matter. Our work on the base mattered. The woman earning the Purple Heart after combat matters. It's all connected. And even though one single study alone could not change history, even though we provided one more piece of evidence in a pile of military research proving the power of women, even though we might not have directly caused the changes, had we *failed*, our poor results would have added to the other basket—we'd have provided a reason *not* to open up combat jobs to females. That was never going to happen on our watch. As Eric put it recently, "Your study was one of a kind."

And so history was made by a group of women they called ordinary. It took a bartender, a beautician, a lawyer, a reporter, a stay-at-home mom, a landscaper, a student, a working mom, an entrepreneur, a prison guard and a teacher to get us that much closer to recognizing the power of women. In the final test, we discovered the most valuable lesson of all: That victory is not always in the winning, but in the conduct, and when it was over we knew we truly were in a league of our own.

16

Back for good

I knew about the study's journey, and now it was time to track down the women who made it possible. Twenty-four years after that first trek, I started searching for the friends I'd adored so but had lost in the tailwinds of fast, turbulent decades. On a cool October day in 2019 I reconnected with Nadine. She'd started a new business and lived in a purple house in Ashland, a quiet New England suburb twenty-eight miles west of Boston. I'd forgotten her attachment to the color purple, forgotten that if you knew Nadine, a shade of Concord grape would be in your life in some form.

"Do you remember?" she asked when we began to compare memories. "Remember what we used to do when someone was stuck out there in the woods?"

I did. Nadine, who after the study had sent me purple-themed birthday cards until she lost track of my address after my third move in as many years, brought the memories back into sharp relief, painting a vintage picture of our unspoken battle cry back then: *No woman left behind.* That autumn I contacted everyone whose full names I could remember—many had changed with marriage, and there were some women from A, B and D groups whose last names I never knew—and whose contact details I could dig up. Most of us lost touch within a few years after the study ended, partly because there was no social media back then, but also because there was barely *email* in 1995.

I wrote emails and poked social media pages and snail-mailed cards. One by one I found them, and as I spoke to my old friends and saw them over FaceTime or in person, it was as if no time had passed. I realized then we'd been given the rare gift of *not* keeping in touch, spared the cherry picked pieces of a life in filtered, curated images populating the unreal landscape of social media. We'd said goodbye when the study came to a close and then met up again at the other end of the wormhole. The years between 1995 and 2020 were one blink of an eye, a whisper in time, a promise in four words: *I'll see you later.* So much else had changed, but our experiences together were preserved in amber inside our hearts and minds.

As our beloved trainer, the funny, talented, supportive, heartless, brutal and performance-minded Eric told me when he and I reconnected, "That study was so unique. I worked with the Army for eighteen years after that, and I never saw another one like it."

I found Jean, late joiner to C-Group, erstwhile cruise bunkmate and former Toys 'R' Us worker bee, back at the Labs. Not long after the study, she built a career in finance, married and changed her name to Jean Trumpis, had two children, and as of 2021 works on the Natick post as a program analyst managing the money for various programs and projects. In some ways it was like coming home; in others, she remains acutely aware of her civilian status.

"Working for the Army is different," she says now. "There are certain security measures, but I was already familiar with the location. It felt comfortable coming back." They felt comfortable having her back, too. Not long after she started, someone from the old days approached her. It was John Kirk, the lead engineer for Load Bearing Equipment for what is now the Combat Capabilities Development Command Soldier Center (CCDC).

"So eleven years later, John Kirk comes up to me and says, 'I remember you, you were part of the backpack study I did,'" Jean recalls with amazement. "I couldn't believe he recognized me, I was like, 'that was so long ago!' You remember we graded each of the packs we wore? While we were doing the 75-pound backpack run, they were testing the packs we were using."

Cement Hill is a part of Jean's life again, and she had a bluntly brutal update for me: It was never really that bad. "I see Cement Hill and I think about my 'just fucking do it' attitude," Jean reflects now. "Was it *that* hard? It's not as big, or as long as we thought it was." She has learned to forgive it its trespasses (though to be fair she doesn't have to run up it anymore). "It's really kind of funny to think we hated this hill. It's not that bad."

Jean, now divorced and raising two boys with her ex, invited me onto the base for a walk, and we made loose plans to meet up for lunch and a stroll up our old nemesis, and I started the process of getting Army clearance for a base visit. They say you can never go back, but I was ready to be there again, to see that lake and face Cement Hill. And then the pandemic hit. COVID-19 changed the world in a minute, taking lives, halting future plans and stealing dreams, and we can hope it won't be for much longer as vaccines are approved and start mass production in the study's twenty-fifth anniversary year.

The study helped shape Jean, honed her ability to push through pain, to keep her cool, to never give up. She keeps her newspaper front page on her office wall, forever a reminder of what she accomplished. "I always enjoyed going, I loved working out with you guys," she says. "Even when I was like, 'what the fuck do we have to do this for?' I liked suffering through it with all of you."

Denise LePage lives near the base and has owned her own company, which she markets as "Home of the Ultimate Sport Card Display," for decades. It keeps ticking along while she works in a medical office with benefits "until somebody would love to buy a million units of sports card displays," she half-jokes. The study has been an evergreen metaphor for everything in her life. "I started the company in 1998 and it's still going," she says. "If you want to succeed, you keep working on it, and you get there, just like the backpack test."

Jane Crowley Dunbar married her fiancé shortly after the study. They eventually divorced, and she is now a writer living in Vermont with her longtime partner. Because of the study, she says, she went from loathing running to signing up for marathons, which seemed to her "like an insurmountable goal, but I knew I could do it because I went through the study and what the hell is harder than that? I learned a lot about myself. I can perform at a much higher level than I ever thought I was capable of; I'm pretty strong physically and mentally, and I'd never really thought about myself like that before."

I could hear Donna—now Donna Terestre—smiling through the phone when we reconnected. She was ready to talk openly about all of it, to trust me now as we'd trusted each other so long ago on Cement Hill. I found her happily married in Auburn, Massachusetts and still working in the newspaper business. In my own mind I'd glossed over the fact she'd left C-Group—and so had she. "Until you told me, I'd completely forgotten," she says now in disbelief.

At one of our big parties toward the end of the study, I heard a test subject mention in passing that Donna was in a relationship with a volunteer in another group who was also at that event. I was never sure, and didn't give it much thought; we were there to do a job and the women tended to respect one another's boundaries. Donna wasn't the only one who didn't run around chattering about her life story. To this day I couldn't tell you if Amanda had a serious boyfriend at the time or was divorced or the CEO of a major company; in my memory, she didn't talk much about her personal or professional life, and sadly I was never able to reach her for this book despite calls and letters sent to her last known address.

But now Donna and I talked about her marriage, an enduring one that, she says, makes up fifteen years of their twenty-one-year union. "It wasn't legal for us to be married until then," Donna says. Her wife's name is Cindy. Donna tells me this and suggests I probably never knew, but she is gay, and happy, and child-free.

"Me too," I told her, about the kids part.

"And that's OK," she replied firmly, quickly.

We've both gotten the question for years and still do, I know that for sure, because all women do. The cock of the head; the question asked brightly, expecting a *yes,* and then the scramble to make things less awkward when they hear *no*, but really we're usually quite well, thank you.

"You didn't share that you were in a relationship with a woman with anyone back then?" I asked her.

"Oh, no. I never would've told anyone in 1995. For one thing, I liked Elle a lot, and it would've broken my heart if she cut me off." Those words broke *my* heart. "I definitely held it in. People get funny."

They did get funny then, and they still do, and it's still unfair and completely outrageous and stupid. Yet when Donna and I talk of the close friendships formed back then, she admits to keeping a bit more distance than some of us did. "It's a little bit hard," she says now. "As much as I tried to experience that time to the fullest extent, there was always the big thing I held back. The older I get the more I realize *I* lost out on the close friendships. If I had been more open and honest, I would have gotten more out of it. I didn't keep in touch with people because I didn't want to share that.

"There was another thing, too," she added. "It was the middle of Don't Ask, Don't Tell, and we were on an Army base."

She said it all calmly, while I grew more pissed off at the fundamental unfairness of it. Presumably because she's had to deal with insensitive morons and bigots her entire life, and I had the privilege of never having to explain my love life to anyone. I would ask Elle about Donna's concerns, I decided, if I ever managed to find her.

Donna says the study changed her. She hasn't stopped running since the old days, when she walked away with a home gym and a legacy. "Every once in awhile it comes up, and people are like 'wow, you really did that?' and I'm like 'yeah, I can't believe it now.' It's funny you say we made five-hundred dollars," she laughs. "In my head it was like fifteen hundred. For twenty-five years I thought that. I still use the gym. It's important to me to keep working out. I wanted to keep going after the study. I had lost some weight, I felt fitter, I looked fitter. I didn't want to lose that."

Donna and I ended the call with promises to get together, and I'd meet Cindy and she'd meet my husband, and we'd have a grand old time remembering the good things about 1995. I still have the note she wrote on a card

C-Group gave me referencing how we'd have to dodge bird crap on so many of our runs: *Sara—I know you'll always step around the goose shit of life. Live long and prosper – Donna.*

I met Stacey Coady for Caesar salads and dirty martinis to rehash the good old days. We got right into recalling our common ground, which included a strong distaste for running. She disliked that part of the study as much as I did, yet lives with four track stars—three grown kids and her longtime partner, Eric.

She'd had all the optimism in the world when the study ended, all the opportunity, but says some things didn't turn out as she'd hoped. An exciting start to her law career turned into working on a single case for fifteen years, and despite prevailing against a major Boston law firm, she says the victory "felt hollow" after gaining experience in a profession where, she believes, "sometimes the only true winners are the large firms that receive millions in fees as a reward for losing their side of the case."

Years after she'd set out to prove Newt Gingrich wrong, Stacey found herself once again fighting for young female athletes as her father had back in the seventies. When her daughter reached high school, she became a top track star—and suffered injuries Stacey viewed as preventable in part due to practices being held on the unforgiving surfaces of school hallways. When Stacey tried to bring her concerns to the Wellesley High School athletics department, offering to help find safer alternatives for practices, she says she got nowhere. She stood up at a Town Hall in 2016 and told how she was met "with nothing but resistance and retaliation" when she contacted school officials to problem-solve. Others, including a senior soccer team captain, shared similar experiences. School officials responded and promised to do better. Stacey enrolled her track champion daughter elsewhere, and she thrived.

Stacey, who came to lunch with binders of correspondence between her, the school, and other concerned parents, felt as if she gave everything to make things better for female athletes and changed nothing, and that her daughter suffered for it. "But you did succeed," I said. "Your daughter saw you stand up for girls and women. She saw you fight through it."

"Yeah," Stacey replied wearily. Her daughter is towering and strong and stunning like her mom, and has begun to break into the modeling industry. "She's already been asked to travel to sketchy 'photo shoots.' How do I keep her from predators? How do I tell her that her body is beautiful, yes, but it's who she *is* that matters?"

I had no answer. For women it is still about looks vs. performance, surface vs. character, the male gaze vs. staying true to how *you* want your body to be. "I'm not sure anything's gotten better," Stacey says. "Even with #MeToo. It still feels the same as when we were young." I couldn't entirely disagree. Still, she keeps going, spending time with her family, staying active and, she says, will never stop fighting for what she believes in.

When I left that lunch, one of the last face-to-face interviews I had with any of the test subjects pre-pandemic, a realization hit me: I'd been talking to all these people about the struggle of carrying a 75-lb backpack for two miles, but I hadn't acknowledged to myself that I was still bearing a weight I didn't need, and it came with me everywhere. After the holidays, I slowly, slowly began getting back in touch with my body and what it needed to regulate. I lifted heavier weights more often. I ate fewer meals. Smaller meals. I was back to losing a teaspoon of fat a week, and that was OK, because I would never, ever again obsess over bread or wring my napkin at dinner while everyone else ate dessert or starve myself to distraction. I would find balance above all else.

There were many moments over twenty-five years that I ached to know the ending to my story with Elle. Without answers from her, I'd walked out of the movie just before the big reveal. I'd checked out of New England in 1996 and left my new favorite book behind only three-quarters read.

When I found her online, I emailed her with careful, formal wording, and heard back within hours: *I'm about to leave for vacation but I'm HAPPY to hear from you and I wanted you to know that. More later!* That was the last I heard from her for months. I accepted I'd have to continue guessing what she'd been thinking all these years.

As the book inched closer to completion, I felt a responsibility to make sure Elle had a chance to be included if she wanted to be, and I sent her a final email. Two minutes later my phone rang. The laughing voice I'd written about, the one that announced *Elle* was here, exploded down the phone, and I was instantly laughing too, because we were back in the training room and she was sharing her latest joke or mishap like no time had passed. We chatted about where we were and how our lives turned out—she's running a church in Florida with Macon, now an ordained pastor *and* a business consultant, and has a bunch of kids and grandkids who all live on the same block.

Elle told me there was a reckoning in their marriage as the study ended, and for the next few years while they lived in Massachusetts they readjusted and formed a new incarnation of their relationship. The study had changed them as a couple. Macon was a well-to-do consultant, traveling and helping businesses thrive, and his wife was absorbed by this odd, all-encompassing, soul-excavating experience that by its nature was an exclusive one. I was too (insert adjective: self-absorbed, inexperienced, young) to get what was going on. Elle rarely seemed upset or conflicted. She never bailed on a social event or missed a training session. Macon didn't try to hold her back, and Elle didn't give me any indication that he was anything other than supportive of her adventure.

"Is your husband excited about the study and the book?" she asked me.

"He is," I told her. "He's excited that *I'm* so excited about it. He thinks it sounds cool. But he doesn't entirely get it."

My husband does show a suitable level of enthusiasm, but he's happy for me at a certain distance. He couldn't possibly understand. I told Elle this.

"It's like what you said," Elle reveals now. "I was so deeply involved in the study, meeting new people, making friends. Macon was on the fringes a little bit, and that created a distance. He didn't know the same people. He didn't know what I was going through."

"But you're happy together now?" I asked.

"You know," she said, "I've been married nearly thirty years. Happiness is not a state of being. It's a feeling that comes and goes. Anyone who tells you different isn't being honest. Marriages have their ups and downs, and it's getting through those times that makes it successful."

I once read advice from someone's grandmother: *The best hope you have is that both people don't want to leave the relationship at the same time. As long as one person still wants to make it work, you have a chance.* I told her that's how it's been for me for nineteen years, and she replied, "Yes! That, too."

And then, ice broken and heat slowly kicking on, we felt safe enough to get down to it. "I wasn't sure how you'd feel hearing from me after how it all ended," I told her. "I was acting out. I wasn't very nice. I was immature."

She trailed off, stammered. "Wow. Uh, I want to be honest, but…"

I felt a creeping dread. Did she remember me as despicably horrible and angry? Or forgivably, understandably hurt? Or somewhere in between?

"We're all being real in this book," I replied. "You can say anything."

She took a breath, and then confessed, "I *don't remember*. I had no memory of a falling out. When you contacted me, I was just happy."

I wasn't insulted the way she thought I would be; I was

relieved I hadn't reacted so outrageously that the negativity stuck with her. She asked me to recap, and I told her everything. I felt silly saying it aloud, but I let it all out, reminded her how we left things, and told her why I was hurt.

She responded softly, "Oh, my. I'm sorry. I'm so sorry I did that. I'm sorry I didn't recognize it as the big thing that it was. I don't know if somebody asked me to room with them, and I probably just said 'sure!' I love people and I was probably clueless…and worse. I don't want anyone to be left out or locked out ever. I struggle with people being left out. I have my entire life."

In every pause, I was uttering *It's fine it's fine it's ok it doesn't matter now, no big deal.* I said sorry to her, too, but the apology dissolved on its way out of my mouth. She says she doesn't remember anything I need to be sorry for. I *was* sorry, though, for being dark after everything changed with us. I *wasn't* sorry for being hurt and separating myself from her.

Elle and her sprawling brood now spend hours in church and their downtime at the beach, where Elle's youngest child plays in the surf with her grandchildren—one of Elle's kids is the same age as little Mona's child. Mona, the little girl who had hope and admiration in her voice as she yelled to us, "Run, mommy, run!" on the base on those summer days, is now a wife, mother and teacher.

Elle brought God up a few times in our chat, and relayed how much her faith directs her life. "God gave you every gift there is that you need to be the success he created you to be," she told me, and then uttered a version of the "I'm no better than anyone else, and no worse" she'd said on the base in 1995. She adds now, "If you really think about it, once you really, truly believe you are no worse than anyone else, you are free. If you had felt that way when I roomed with someone else, you wouldn't have felt so hurt."

I can't agree entirely on that last assumption, but she had a point. I asked her about Donna then. I told her exactly what our friend said to me about begin afraid to tell. "Oh, no!" Elle responded. "I wondered if she thought that. No, no, *no*. I adore her."

Regardless of how Elle and I ended, and how different we are, the study remains a thread connecting us. Elle talked about how she remembered me, and she said, "You were always brave and beautiful. You know you are."

No one has called me brave or beautiful in so long, I told her. I asked her how the study affected her. She spoke of emotional and physical strength, of friendships, of precious memories, and the value of pushing yourself past your limits. "The times you succeed are not when you played it safe," Elle says. "They're when you put yourself out there and try your hardest. You have to put some risk into it."

Elle gave me the ending I'd craved. I'm not sure how much she and I have in common or ever did or how much our world views are aligned, but the study will connect us forever, and I'm glad I knew her.

I prayed Marion was alive. I had dark thoughts as I imagined what might've befallen her in the line of duty, and

I fretted that I hadn't kept in touch. I realized this person I'd once called a best friend was serving our country in danger zones while I was running around chasing Tom Cruise and Jennifer Aniston—and making no effort to find out how Marion was. Not that she needed me to, but twenty-four years after the fact seemed too little, too late to check on a "friend's" well-being.

I thought about Billy, too. When it came time to look for them, I was less worried about Marion than I was about Billy. I knew she wouldn't have been welcome on the frontlines, in battle, in the trenches. While the combat policies didn't keep women out of danger, particularly medics, it surely reduced the odds, I figured. I also thought about the depression that could've continued to hurt my friend.

I found Marion on Facebook, sent a friend request, and heard nothing. I still didn't know if she was alive. And then, one day, on my own barely used Facebook page, I saw that beautiful red notification: Marion had accepted my request. Spoiler alert: She was fine. It took three more weeks to connect via email, and then another three months to connect via phone, and then finally, in one laughter-filled, cathartic evening, we reunited on FaceTime. There wasn't a whiff of awkwardness or pause. She and I, alone in our separate rooms in separate states, were back in 1995 together, and our phones were the DeLoreans whisking us there. The delay in connecting, it turned out, had been due to an epic life change: I'd found her just two weeks after she'd ended her twenty-five-year Army career. It was a great relief to find Marion in one piece, thriving even, still living around Fort Bragg in North Carolina.

With all the talk of the nineties and fitness, we quickly got to pining for our twenty-something physiques, and Marion recalled how much she was running and working out even outside of our study. “It wasn’t this obsessive thing,” she remembers. “I was in great shape, but it was more about performance with what we were doing, not looks. By the time it was over, I was in the best shape of my life. Can you believe we didn’t appreciate our bodies then? Why did we ever complain about how we looked? Wouldn’t you give anything to be in that kind of shape again?”

No and *Hell yes*, I replied to two of her questions. There were no barriers to real talk, and we dissected the past, fitness, weight, aging, men, children (she is contentedly child-free), and how life turned out. Marion, who continues to work on managing her mental health, has never forgotten C-Group rallying around her when her depression first hit. “I can visualize all of you that day,” Marion says of the moment she revealed her struggle. “I can see in my head where it was outside, what corner of the building it was, and you all were talking to me. You and Elle both said, ‘you need to do something. Go see a doctor.’ Those were the times before everybody was going to see somebody and taking medication and whatever. It was you all who convinced me to do it.”

Her new civilian friends, all older than her, some of us almost like aunts, formed a cocoon. “I remember loving all you guys, and that the study was like a safe space or whatever we would have called it then," she says. "That's a newer term, but we were all good friends and we told each other everything. And I didn't feel any sense of judgment."

Marion left our study in 1995 a walking prototype for Ev's program as she launched into her next Army posting. "It was like CrossFit before there was CrossFit," she says. "I think it kind of prepared me for anything. Not one specific task, necessarily, but for any sort of physical feat and activity. We were all really well balanced at the end for strength, kinetic energy, ruck marching, running.

"After Natick, I went to air assault school, and that was physically easy for me. At the very end you have to do a twelve-mile ruck march, I don't remember the weight, but I was running with this other girl and we got our calculations wrong—we thought we were behind, so we went harder and faster, and then we figured out we were *way* ahead."

In another stroke of serendipity for Marion and Billy, both were sent to Korea for their next posting and managed to squeeze in time for a backpacking trip around Europe before shipping out. Things were good then, but once they arrived in Korea their relationship was tested. Says Marion, "He was up on the DMZ and really isolated."

The close couple became on-again-and-off-again, she says. Before long, they were separated not only by a rocky relationship, but by geography. "It was 2000 when I went to Kosovo," she tells me. "We did a lot of development with the NGO community, local leaders, and different programs."

Marion was on leave when the 9/11 attacks happened, and she was sent to Iraq as the war began. I, a person who is afraid of heights and spiders, asked her how fearful she was go to into the hot zone. Marion wasn't technically allowed into combat in the early 2000s, but as a medic she would still likely end up on frontlines of some description. "I wasn't scared," she told me. "I don't think I was nervous. It was just what you did."

Marion and I talked about the other risks females in our military face. Sexism, misogyny, harassment and sexual assault are the enemies within. In 2019, the U.S. military fielded 7,825 sexual assault reports among service members and 1,021 formal sexual harassment complaints, according to a DOD report. Fort Hood Soldier Vanessa Guillen's case catapulted the issue into the public consciousness once again in 2020 after she disappeared and tragically was later found dead. Her family believes she was sexually harassed by a senior officer but was terrified of retribution if she reported it, and her case sparked a fresh national conversation about sexual harassment and assault in the military. Some have used that unacceptable scourge as an argument to keep women out of infantry, special forces, and combat. But the solution is the opposite move, many others argue: what better way to chip away at that toxic culture than to elevate more women to higher ranks? There seems a far greater chance of eliminating harassment and assault with female bosses in place to scrape the rot from the inside out.

Like all the military women I've spoken with over the

years, Marion developed skin like armor, though she never should've had to. And that armor had its vulnerabilities. The worst it got for her was in Iraq, where she was a staff sergeant in the U.S. Army Reserve.

"At first I was the only woman in my company, until one girl, my roommate, got moved, so she ended up coming to Sulaymaniyah where we were stationed," she recalls. "There were some hard parts, just getting harassed and being judged on everything I did. I could never get the same credit for doing the same thing as one of the guys. It was always considered less. That's been my whole career. Guys aren't judged like that; women are immediately judged and you're considered lesser until you prove yourself. I still don't totally know what the deal was—it was just kind of really unhappy asshole guys looking to lash out and show their dominance." Most of her team, she adds, had her back and would step in if they saw her being harassed.

After leaving Iraq she moved on to Fort Bragg, where she was eventually assigned to an exciting new military program that had been launched in 2010. Although qualified women still could not even attempt to join special ops teams such as the Army Rangers or Navy SEALs, the U.S. Army Special Operations Command came up with a way to bring women in on the periphery. Dubbed the Cultural Support Teams (CST) pilot program, the new approach exploited certain vague language in the 1994 combat exclusion rule that allowed women to be "attached" to special ops teams going into combat. Working mostly in pairs of two, the female teams would accompany elite male units on sensitive missions and build bridges and relationships with local residents so the special ops guys—like Rangers and SEALS—could coax life-saving intel from villagers who would never, could never, speak to a strange man.

Make no mistake: The women were in harm's way right alongside the men. Not long after the program's inception, on Oct. 22, 2011, First Lieutenant Ashley White-Stumpf, who was embedded with the Army's 75th Ranger Regiment, was killed by an improvised explosive device in Afghanistan's Kandahar province during a night raid (her story has been told with great care in *Ashley's War* by Gayle Tzemach Lemmon). White-Stumpf was posthumously awarded medals including the Bronze Star, the Purple Heart, and the Combat Action Badge.

Marion was named CST program manager in 2012. Her group would be assigned to the elite Army Rangers and special forces, and they would be put through a punishing training regimen known as "100 hours of hell."

"I got their applications, and I remember sitting down and opening the first file on one of these women, and I was like, holy *shit* this girl's a badass," Marion remembers. "And I opened the next one and I was like *damn*. It was one after the other. We didn't look for a specific age, but we looked for different iterations in backgrounds. The oldest I worked with was forty-one, but that's an anomaly. Most were in their late twenties.

"I was always really proud of them. They were pretty much all elite, strong women. They weren't just strong physically, but mentally. They go through this assessment selection and they're chosen for certain traits. You had cream-of-the-crop females from across the military—we had some from the Air Force, too—so it was really nice to see because they did go in and prove themselves worthy, and I think for a lot of guys that was their first time working with women. The men would be skeptical, but they would see the value of having women and a lot of them ended up asking for more of them for missions."

Sadly, Marion would experience the full spectrum of success and tragedy as program manager. First Lieutenant Jennifer Moreno was killed on Oct. 6, 2013, after an IED blast three months into her first deployment with the Army's 75th Ranger Regiment. Two Army Rangers, Sergeant Patrick C. Hawkins and Private First Class Cody J. Patterson, and Army Special Agent Joseph M. Peters also died. In addition to receiving a Bronze Star Medal, Moreno was posthumously promoted to captain.

"She ran to save people," Marion told me of the young woman she'd gotten to know. "She helped people in the blast. She was so young. The thing I remember most about her is she always had the biggest smile, that kind of big cheeky smile; you'd never see her without that smile. That's how she looked all the time. She was a really sweet girl. She had a teammate who was especially affected. She's still very close to Jennifer's family."

Marion, too, was grief-stricken. "When it happened, I found out when her funeral was, and I went in to my commander and asked if I could go to the funeral in California. Before I even finished asking, he was like, *Yes.*

And he made sure I got orders and it got paid for and to me that was so important; still to this day I need to thank him again.

"We got really close. To this day some of those girls are my good friends. They would refer to themselves as 'our band of sisters.' And that really was good to see. These are very high performing women, but they are for the most part not negatively competitive; they make each other better and they're all very supportive of each other. Saying 'woman power' might seem lame and cliché, but they still network for each other and help each other succeed."

Marion eventually said goodbye to the CST and went to work for a surgeon's office covering special operations training. She stuck with that for three years until she retired from the military for good and went on to pursue a degree in global public health at the University of North Carolina, Chapel Hill.

When we got off the phone after nearly three hours, I was ready to search for Billy. All I hoped for was to find him alive, somewhere out there walking around, still grinning. And so he is. Major Billy Wade lives in the deep south and is married with children, is no longer a medic, and works in several arenas of our country's defense, including electronic warfare.

I had said goodbye to the boy in 1995 and twenty-five years later I met the man when we caught up by phone. His southern twang is even stronger now, and he is as polite as ever. Like the rest of us from that time on the Natick base, he was hit with a wave of nostalgia as we recalled the old days. "Those times were honestly, still to this day, some of the best memories of my life," he said. "I always loved Boston and Natick and that time; that was me transitioning from boy to man. I was doing a really cool job for the military that not many people get to do, and I met a lot of cool people. I stayed in touch with a lot of them and I still do. It was a great time in my life. Everyone I met there I would consider a friend."

I asked him if he remembered our box lift test, and I told him I was nervous about beating his score but had been pleasantly surprised by his reaction. His reply came with the same calm acceptance he'd shown decades before when I'd beaten him: "I was raised by my sister and my mom. My dad was around but he was gone a lot. I never felt any worse or any better from anybody, male or female. People are better at certain things—you can't win at everything."

As hard as he's worked over the years, he's never taken his varied experiences for granted. "It's been a fun ride," he told me. "I've been so many places. I've played music in the streets with gypsies. I try to play music wherever I go."

A few months after my first reunion with Marion, as the coronavirus was ravaging every corner of the world, I checked in with her, texting an adorable photo of us I'd dug up. She wrote back, *I love us!... Volunteering at a food bank. I'll update you soon...Miss ya! Love ya!* Of *course* she was volunteering. She'd just left the Army, but she couldn't stop serving, and mid-pandemic she was risking her own health to feed people in need.

There are periods in a life we all romanticize, but with the study, there was no denial or glossy filter brightening our memories. It was all perfect *because* of its torments and tears and missteps, its freckles and warts and tears.

Eric flew his own way after the study ended, spread his wings, and took on the exciting projects the Army assigned him. Mary focused on her career and her master's degree in Boston. They stayed together through the unsettling shift in schedules; their bond was tight and Mary is a patient, secure woman. Eventually, Eric began to spend more time in Massachusetts and, says Mary, "our relationship grew from there." Before long, she was ready to talk about marriage—but Eric remained hesitant.

"He needed a bit of nudging in the marriage department," Mary recalls. "He's fearless in so many ways but when it came to this, not so much. I think he was afraid marriage would clip his wings. I was able to show him he didn't need to choose. We could have both."

She told him, and he listened. "I never saw myself settling down, but the more time Mary and I spent together, the more it seemed possible to me," Eric says. "It was a revelation I wasn't expecting. We began traveling together to Europe, climbed mountains in the Tetons, and have done numerous treks in the Swiss Alps. And at the same time we were building a life together back in Massachusetts."

In the end, he chose Mary over his fear of commitment. They tied the knot in November of 2001, two months after

I got married fifty miles from them. There was soon talk of kids; Mary had always wanted children. Again Eric took a leap of faith with her.

"When we got pregnant, we were happy but scared at the same time," Mary recalls. "What were we supposed to do with a *baby*? We had done so many amazing things together pre-kids, and I think we were both worried that this would change who we were. It definitely did—but in the best way possible."

They are parents to two teens now, a boy and a girl. "I never would in a million years have guessed he would be the kind of dad he is," says Mary, who's now Assistant Superintendent for Student Support Services in a Massachusetts school system. "Eric's so committed. He's 110 percent in. As my jobs got more intense over the years, gradually he went from working full time, to part time, to picking up some coaching positions, and essentially he's been a stay-at-home dad for the last several years. He does everything: lunches, pick up and drop off, and dinner."

"I thought having a family would change things, and it has," Eric adds. "Now we just do all of the things we love *together*—like traveling, skiing, hiking and camping."

During one of our recent conversations, he asked me, "Why don't you have kids?" After a pause, he added, "If you don't mind me asking."

He had every right to expect me to be as honest as I was asking everyone else in this book to be. I told him it hadn't worked out for us, though we tried, and then I reeled off the good things about not having them, of which there are many. Not everyone gets everything. He replied, "Before I had kids, I couldn't understand why people did it. After, I can't understand why people don't. It makes you do things you otherwise wouldn't. Like—you go cross-country skiing when you might not otherwise."

He's not wrong. I don't go cross-country skiing if I don't have to.

Mary says the pair has the same important things in common now as they did twenty-five years ago. "When I think about how life gets on fast forward, it's so busy now," she says. "It used to be breakfast, but some of the quiet times for us are at night now. I work long days and have a lot of evening commitments, I'll get home around seven, and he's cooked dinner and done all the homework, and we'll have dinner as a family. And the teenagers take off, so Eric and I will have a few minutes at the table just chatting. That reminds me of what it was like when we first met. We have these slivers of time and that's when we can talk about anything, big life things, or, currently, it's about the bathtub leaking upstairs and he's trying to figure out how to fix it."

Laughing now at the old days when he moved in with his camping pad and javelin and, later, a cardboard chest of drawers, Mary says, "To this day he doesn't want a lot or need a lot. I'm different than that; I like a nice house and actual furniture, so we've built a good marriage around compromise."

Chris Palmer is now a high-flying consultant and boasts a twenty-five-year career working in various capacities for the Department of Defense. He has two adult children—a son and a daughter—and lives in Massachusetts with his wife and daughter. Ev left USARIEM in 2008 and began focusing more on the fitness aspect of his expertise than on science, starting a wellness blog for men and religiously keeping up his own workouts. He met someone new along the way, got married again, and has three more kids (for a total of five) who keep him young; I see him all over social media taking them on hikes and on adventures and showing friends and family how they're excelling in academics.

Pete continues to love his job solving problems for the military on the Natick base. "When I hear people say they're bored, I think, *You're not paying attention*," he says now. "There are too many amazing things out there to ever be bored in this world." Outside of work, Pete spends his downtime beekeeping. When we met up again, he gave us all little bear-shaped jars of his honey, and told me, "I'm studying to be a master beekeeper now. Bees are endlessly fascinating. Each hive will have 40,000 bees in it. Every third bite of food you eat is directly pollinated by an insect. Now I live with a wife, a dog, chickens in the yard, and at the peak of the season a quarter of a million bees, so it's all females all the time."

Catherine: 2020

I first spoke to Catherine in the winter of 2019 when she was two-thirds of the way through her next course, this time at Twentynine Palms, California. It was the last stop for Second Lieutenant Afton before embarking on her career as a Marine officer. Her first billet would be assigned at the end, and if she shone, she could have her pick of plum assignments. Far from being fatigued from all that came before, I found her raring to go and intending to finish first. At the time, number one and number two in the class—rankings that take into account physical and academic achievements—were both women: Catherine and a good friend of hers.

This course was about learning the technical aspects of her future job (MOS) in logistics, and throughout it Catherine hovered among the top three in her class. And then, as the end neared, she figured out what she wanted—a posting in in Asia. Problem was, she was being offered a U.S. post, albeit in a sun-drenched locale. "It was a decision I had to make," she remembers. "They said, 'You have twenty-four hours—go.'"

Easier said than done. Catherine had a schedule so packed that sleep was an afterthought. "I was planning to run the Marine Corps marathon in D.C. on the Sunday, but my school schedule kept shifting around," she recalls of those key days. "I thought it would be fine, but then it ended up that Monday and Tuesday I was in charge of planning this whole big presentation, and our redeye left Friday from Vegas.

"I almost told my friend, 'I don't know if I can do it.' But then I thought, of *course* I want to do it. What better way to test myself? We drove three hours to Vegas, took a redeye, slept on Saturday, ran on Sunday. The night the decision was due was the night of the marathon, and I was running the whole marathon thinking about it." Not long after she crossed the finish line, "I took another two flights back, then drove to Twentynine Palms, took an hour nap, and had to plan a whole exercise—I had to give a speech with forty slides including diagrams."

I was staggered by the story, told almost as speedily as it must have unfolded, in part maybe because I forgot what it was like to be young and bounce back. I asked her how she handles that kind of stress. "Nah," she replied. "It's low stress, because if I mess up it's not real. If I mess up I wouldn't be taking peoples lives."

So said the woman about to embark on her first assignment as a working Marine Corps officer. She was not afraid of her first real job, though she couldn't have known her career would launch amid a global pandemic. "All my friends will be overseas, so that's hard," she told me. "But here I'll have a voice and my voice matters, and if I know what I'm talking about, I'll be fine. I'll have a platoon. I'll have twenty-five Marines and millions of dollars in equipment." She paused, shrugged. "I'm going to get yelled at so much."

Catherine graduated a close third to her friend and a guy. It had been an honorable race, with each pushing the other to strive for number one. "Three of us were within reach. None of us said until the last week that we all wanted it," she says now.

Her mother had wanted to fly out to Twentynine Palms and watch her graduate, but Catherine downplayed the event. It was more a ceremony within their own world than a spectacle for loved ones. It wasn't necessary, Catherine told her mom. She flew home afterward and took a bus to the suburbs, and when she stepped onto the familiar ground of her hometown, Catherine saw her mom waiting there with a grand smile. My friend Nadine opened her arms and embraced the daughter she'd missed so. She peppered the exhausted Marine with questions on the ride home to the purple house, and once there, Catherine greeted the family and then slept for a long, long time.

Nadine has always believed that Catherine's unstoppable drive, her particular way of running toward pain, began in the womb. "It is another amazing thing about that study," Nadine says now, "that my daughter's trajectory in life is *because* of it. I'm convinced she's a Marine because while I was pregnant with her I was doing the study, and that was *all* that was on my mind. All I thought about was accomplishing it and doing it, and like me, Catherine had set her sights very young on succeeding.

"I have four children. In many ways the bond I had with Catherine was strong because of the competitiveness we both have. One summer a few years ago, I was doing sit-ups. I did twenty-five, and she said, 'that's nothing. I can do fifty.' She does fifty and I'm like, 'you little shit, I can do sixty.' We went about this every week that summer, and I got up to 1,025 and she did 1,041 and I said, 'that's it. I fold, I fold.'

"My other kids I didn't have that with. None of them care about the challenge the way she and I do. It's interesting. The whole structure of the study was about using that skillset of mind over matter, and never giving up." (Side note: We also talked about her other three children's unique gifts and personalities, but they wanted to remain anonymous).

Added Nadine of that pregnancy that threw Eric on the day she ran by him, "I felt bad my data technically couldn't be used, I regretted that, but that was the deal. I was thinking, what harm can it possibly be? I'm going to be able to deliver a kid with no medicine, in such great shape."

This staunch belief that the Natick strength study created Catherine the Marine perhaps defies logic and science, or maybe there's something to it. Catherine was growing inside Nadine that day in 1995 while she strapped on a creaky 110-pound wagon, keeping her promise to pull it as fast as she possibly could no matter the obstacles. Catherine was there with Nadine as she gutted it out in those woods. Is it so impossible to believe Nadine's current state of being became a part of Catherine in the womb? A mother knows. A mother's instinct can't be discounted.

The daughter Nadine carried now looks upon her with a new layer of respect. Catherine didn't imagine her mother doing such things because it was a long-ago compartment of our life, one summer of the seventy-five or so we're given if we're lucky. "It was fascinating to hear about," Catherine, who was soon promoted to First Lieutenant, says. "I didn't really know about the study until college, once I was in the Marine Corps, or at least that's when I began to understand it; before that, the military wasn't on my radar. Once I knew what she did, I was like *wow*—she has done similar things to what I will do. The coolest part was my mom said they ended up proving we can do what men do. It just might take more time to train us."

As her children fly the coop now one by one, Nadine continues her entrepreneurial efforts as well as her heavy involvement in community building and giving those who need it a leg-up. She still sells insurance. "I'm doing the parts I love, the selling, the connecting with people and keeping in touch over the years," she says. "I get to know who's having a baby, who's going to school, all these great things. As you get older you look at what's good and isn't so good about what you're doing." She started another business, a marketing company called We're All in This Together (WAITT), with the goal of connecting businesses to the community. Her members give a portion of their proceeds to local community organizations.

I wrote the character of Catherine Afton before I knew she existed. I sat down to sketch out what our story might look like on the page even before I contacted any other test subjects, and I started with a screenplay. I conjured a young Marine who attends her graduation while a woman from C-Group, her mother, looks on. I imagined the daughter was benefitting directly from the barriers broken down by the mother. I thought about what an incredible story that would be, an allegory of how much each of us matters, and why it's worth the sacrifice to be the change you want to see; why it's admirable to be the one who plants the tree whose branches you will never sit under.

"The issue we were working on was bigger than just

accomplishing those goals during the tests," Nadine says now. "It was about opening the door to allow my daughter to be a Marine and select combat if she wanted, and I was hoping she didn't want that, but the principle was to open the door."

I was to meet Catherine in person for the first time a few weeks after she left Twentynine Palms. Nadine hosted us at her house, and when I arrived, Nadine went to fetch drinks while I went to freshen up in her bathroom. When I returned to the living room, a young woman was stepping through the opposite doorway ten feet across from me. She was slender with big brown eyes and thick, dark hair falling over one shoulder, and as I clapped eyes on her I was sent back to 1995. My confused brain quite literally took me there for a brief moment while I processed that this was Nadine's daughter, and it took me another few moments to snap back into 2019. For those seconds, I was looking at Nadine walking into a party at Elle's house, and I was twenty-four years old.

Catherine had talked to me about her bonding with other women in training, and how crucial it was to her success, so I asked her to describe what her goodbyes were like at Twentynine Palms. How many graduation banquets did they have? How much pomp, how much circumstance? How many tears were shed in this most important transition in their young lives, in the moments before they would step into the fog of the unknown?

"I've learned there's no such thing as goodbyes," Catherine replied. "I said a lot of goodbyes at TBS and

OCS, and then I saw all those people again. Now it's always 'I'll see you later.' After graduation I didn't stick around for pictures. I just left. There was no goodbye dinner, and I didn't want one."

She looked to her mother, relaxed in a plush chair, and then she turned back to me. "Look at you two," Catherine said. "See? There really is no goodbye."

Nadine and I smiled at each other across the room as the generation after us spoke her truth from a place we could have only dreamed about twenty-five years before, and we were reminded again of why we'd gone through the agony of the study. When I left that night, I hugged Nadine and said to her, "I'll see you later."

Because I know now that I will.

Acknowledgments

Without my friend and visionary Everett Harman, there would be no study, we wouldn't have had this incredible experience, and I wouldn't have had an extraordinary start to my journalism career. He was our calm, guiding force and I am thankful to him for the opportunity beyond measure, and for his help with this book both with interviews and offering valuable feedback on the manuscript. I would not have ever met him or joined his study without Andrea Haynes, an editor ahead of her time who, along with the paper's publisher, had faith in me and let me run with this, and it's time I thanked her again for that.

To Chris, Eric and Pete, who became our friends and our support, who watched us fall and lifted us back up, who showed up every day to help us get strong inside and out, who gave generously of their time and knowledge for this book, THANK YOU. To the amazing, kick-ass women who trusted me to tell their stories without a second's hesitation, there are no words. Catherine, Denise, Donna, Jane, Jean, Laurie, Marion, Mary, Nadine, Shannon, Stacey C., as well as the test subjects who could not be named here: You all inspired me and uplifted me every time we talked. To *all* the women of the Natick Strength Study: This is for you. For however long you were able to stay in it, whether for hours or weeks or months, you did something incredible.

For everyone at the newspaper who supported me and helped create and craft the stories and headlines and images, thank you: From Rus to Doc to Gene and Tom and Jan and especially Ken, whose photographs documented that incredible time. To the gang who picked up the slack and made it fun, you know who you are, especially my friend Rebecca—you are so missed and you are always in my heart. To the friends who helped edit me and advised me on my cover and saved me from myself, like Laurie Anne and Meredyth, thank you. And finally, to my mom for encouraging me to do the study in the first place. For my family. For Chris, for his patience and listening to me process the writing of this book for more than two years, *thank you.*

To those doing the important work for women everywhere who gave me their time and told about the part they played in history, former Secretary of Defense Leon Panetta, Monica Medina, Congresswoman Patricia Schroeder and Shannon Faulkner, I thank you all. It was an honor to include your perspective here. Once again, to our active military and our veterans, THANK YOU.

Sara Hammel

January 1, 2021

The Final Report

1. Harman, E, Frykman, P, Palmer, C, Lammi, E, Reynolds, K, and Backus, V. Effects of a specifically designed physical conditioning program on the load carriage and lifting performance of female soldiers. *Technical Report T98-1.* Natick, MA: US Army Research Institute of Environmental Medicine, 1997.

CPSIA information can be obtained
at www.ICGtesting.com
Printed in the USA
LVHW111936110221
679098LV00036B/539

9 780578 794327